Rehabilitation Counselling

Approaches in the field of disability

Edited by SHARON E. ROBERTSON

Associate Professor
Counselling Psychology Programme
Faculty of Education, University of Calgary, Alberta, Canada

and

ROY I. BROWN

Professor and Director
Rehabilitation Studies Programme
Faculty of Education, University of Calgary, Alberta, Canada

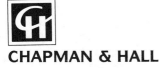

CHAPMAN & HALL
London · Glasgow · New York · Tokyo · Melbourne · Madras

Published by Chapman & Hall, 2–6 Boundary Row, London SE1 8HN

Chapman & Hall, 2–6 Boundary Row, London SE1 8HN, UK

Blackie Academic & Professional, Wester Cleddens Road, Bishopbriggs, Glasgow G64 2NZ, UK

Chapman & Hall, 29 West 35th Street, New York NY10001, USA

Chapman & Hall Japan, Thomson Publishing Japan, Hirakawacho Nemoto Building, 6F, 1-7-11 Hirakawa-cho, Chiyoda-ku, Tokyo 102, Japan

Chapman & Hall Australia, Thomas Nelson Australia, 102 Dodds Street, South Melbourne, Victoria 3205, Australia

Chapman & Hall India, R. Seshadri, 32 Second Main Road, CIT East, Madras 600 035, India

Distributed in the USA and Canada by Singular Publishing Group Inc., 4284 41st Street, San Diego, California 92105

First edition 1992

© 1992 Chapman & Hall

Printed in Great Britain by St Edmundsbury Press Ltd, Bury St Edmunds, Suffolk

ISBN 0 412 36170 1   1 56593 0177 (USA)

9c Acc.No 441/Cat 95/0002847 T
£14.99

REHABILITATION COUNSELLING

This book is to be returned on or before
the last date stamped below.

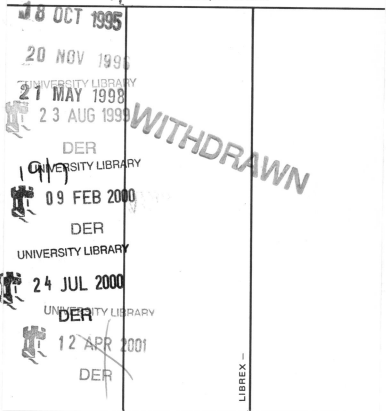

REHABILITATION EDUCATION: A SERIES IN
DEVELOPMENTAL HANDICAP

Edited by Roy I. Brown, University of Calgary

CONTENTS

ACKNOWLEDGEMENTS

The design, development and editing of this book has been the joint responsibility of the two editors. Each chapter has received a detailed edit from one of us, and a second edit with suggested changes from the other editor. After receiving responses from authors on these changes, a final edit has been carried out jointly by both of us. We would like to thank the chapter authors for responding positively to our suggestions, and for carrying out the changes efficiently. The content is from different countries and from people with different backgrounds. We have attempted as editors to keep the philosophical integrity of each chapter. Sometimes there is overlap of content, but we believe that this reflects some of the communalities held across different disciplines, as well as reflecting some of the comparative trends in different settings and various countries.

We wish to thank Kathryn Nikolaychuk for carrying out the initial typing of the manuscript, and also Pat Tempro for completing this process, which involved a change in word processing systems. Her patience in dealing with the issues that arose from this, and bringing to our attention a wide range of printing, is much appreciated. We would also like to thank John Kordyback who was responsible for setting the figures, and for providing advice in relation to technical production of the final copy. Finally, we acknowledge the support of Ms. Terri Cooper of Chapman and Hall, who has provided us with latitude in terms of timing, but has remained encouraging of the final process that led to this text.

S.E.R.
R.I.B.
1991

PREFACE

This is the fifth volume in the Rehabilitation Education Series. It is the second volume to be co-edited, and like its predecessor, concerning Early Intervention, deals with a wide range of issues concerned with disabilities. As the series has developed a much broader perspective has been taken regarding the area of Rehabilitation Education. In this particular volume, the accent on education models and their contribution to the field of rehabilitation, is stressed. In particular, rehabilitation counselling is seen particularly, though not entirely, within this domain. Rehabilitation counselling brings together a wide range of knowledge and skill useful to both professional counsellors and other rehabilitation practitioners as they carry out their day to day business in community and agency.

An attempt has been made to look at generic aspects of disability and examine the social network, particularly the families of people with disabilities. Some considerable stress has been placed on the increasing role that people with disabilities play in deciding the nature of the rehabilitation system, and their particular choices regarding intervention, which are increasingly set within the domain of empowerment. Again, the issues of quality of life have been pursued, and the present speaks to this issue from a wider perspective than in a previous volume, reflecting the growing interest and knowledge in this field as it affects rehabilitation counselling.

S.E.R.
R.I.B.
1991

LIST OF CONTRIBUTORS

Dr. Hy Day
Department of Psychology
York University
4700 Keele Street
North York, Ontario
M3J 1P3 Canada

Drs. Kenneth R. Thomas and
    Randall M. Parker
Department of Therapeutic
    Science
School of Education
University of
    Wisconsin-Madison
1080 Medical Science Center
1300 University Avenue,
Madison, Wisconsin 53706
United States
and
Rehabilitation Counselor
    Education Program
University of Texas at Austin
Austin, Texas
United States

Dr. James W. Vargo
Faculty of Rehabilitation
    Studies
University of Alberta
3 - 48 Corbett Hall
Edmonton, Alberta
T6G 2G4 Canada

Dr. Keith F. Kennett
School of Education
University of Western Sydney
Nepean
P. O. Box 10
Kingswood NSW 2747
Australia

Dr. Sharon E. Robertson
Educational Psychology
The University of Calgary
2500 University Dr. N.W.
Calgary, Alberta
T2N 1N4 Canada

Dr. Gary Hornby
Education Department
University of Hull
Cottingham Road
Hull HU6 7RX
United Kingdom

Susan W. Webb
Massey University
Palmerston North
New Zealand

Dr. Michael J. Holosko
Social Work
University of Windsor
401 Sunset Avenue
Windsor, Ontario
N9B 3P4 Canada

Dr. Gunnel Backenroth
Department of Psychology
Stockholm University
5 - 106 91 Stockholm
Sweden

Dr. Roy I. Brown
Rehabilitation Studies
    Programme
The University of Calgary
2500 University Dr. N.W.
Calgary, Alberta
T2N 1N4 Canada

Chapter One

INTRODUCTION

Roy I. Brown and Sharon E. Robertson

This book represents the fifth volume in the series on rehabilitation education and is particularly concerned with counselling as profession and practice in the field of disability. Consistent with previous volumes, the authors argue for a generic approach towards persons with disabilities believing that the underlying principles from psychological, sociological and ecological perspectives transcend the nature of any specific disability. This does not mean to suggest that there are not differences of levels in application, or different accents required within particular services for particular people, but, rather, there have been unnecessary divisions amongst professionals in provision of services to groups with different disabilities. The theme in this book recognizes the important platform of empowerment by individuals with disabilities, and suggests that the professional skills and procedures that are brought to bear on particular issues generate from individual choices of consumers or clients rather than preconceived notions about needs from professionals. Such a view argues for individualization of approach, and supports a concept of variability amongst groups with different disabilities, thus making any formal or predesignated approach ineffective. It is individuals' notions of their empowerment, their control of choice and their selection of counsellors or practitioners which set the scene for individualized intervention. The training of professionals is much influenced by such a philosophy. The where, how and when of the rehabilitation counsellor's operation is determined by the individual requirements of a specific individual who has a disability.

The field of rehabilitation is a broad one indeed. The United Nations World Programme of Action Concerning Disabled Persons (1983), adopted by the U.N. General Assembly in December, 1982, defines the term as follows:

> Rehabilitation means a goal-directed and time-limited process aimed at enabling an impaired person to reach optimum mental, physical and/or social functional level, thus providing her or him with the tools to change her or his own life. (p.3)

Impairments, disabilities, and handicaps can result from injury, disease, or congenital defect. Thus, such wide-ranging conditions as muscular dystrophy, cerebral palsy, diabetes melittus, hypertension, mental handicap, brain injury, mental illness, and orthopaedic disorders fall within the rehabilitation domain. Individuals of various ages from infancy to old age, their families, and their social environments, serve as the focus for rehabilitation efforts while rehabilitation workers cross-disciplines (e.g. psychology, education, social work, medicine). Counselling, in its broadest sense, might be defined as the provision of help by one person to another in order to solve the latter's life problems (Peavy, Robertson, and Westwood, 1982).

Professional counselling attempts to facilitate human change and development through the use of an extensive set of interlocking skills which are based on specialized knowledge, and guided by a philosophical orientation and ethical guidelines. Rehabilitation counsellors specialize in the needs of persons with disabilities.

Counselling skills are often abstract in quality and not easy to define or prescribe. They are therefore frequently seen as less sophisticated than more traditional interventions which may be biochemical or physical and therefore are more readily understood or accepted. Yet communication in the form of counselling can, when poorly employed, cause great harm. When effective it can help to open up new opportunities, increased awareness and empowerment. As such, counselling deserves to be treated with high priority amongst rehabilitation professionals.

Although Rehabilitation Counsellors are expected to have indepth knowledge and experience of counselling processes all of those working in the rehabilitation field need proficient skills in this area. It is our belief that training in counselling techniques should be part of the education of all those who work directly with persons who have disabilities. Such skills are even more important, as we shall see, when rehabilitation is directed towards community living and adaption. The following chapters are therefore, not only directed to professionally trained rehabilitation counsellors, but also expected to be of value to all those working with people who have disabilities, and wish to communicate and provide support as effectively as possible.

The following chapters represent the views and research of a wide range of people concerned with rehabilitation counselling in different countries. The first chapters are particularly directed towards the notion of rehabilitation counselling, its philosophy and practice, including the general precepts and conditions which motivate or develop the thinking of students in this area. As indicated by Hy Day, it is important to recognize which model or models are to be used within rehabilitation counselling. He makes a cogent argument that rehabilitation counselling, using an educational model has very different implications from using a medical or health-oriented model. Thus, in this book, the terms of "consumer" or "client" are generally used rather than "patient", denoting a psychoeducational perspective where empowerment, choice, and control are encouraged. This is not to argue that one model is more correct than another, but to suggest that unless professionals in the field recognize the basis on which rehabilitation counsellors function, there are likely to be diverse opinions on how counselling is applied or works. Even within such broad domains, there are different approaches to counselling. The principles underlining these are discussed by Thomas and Parker, while some of the individualized processes and practical issues are dealt with in Keith Kennett's chapter. Thomas and Parker provide an overview of the major theories of counselling and psychotherapy and vocational development and occupational choice. They outline how rehabilitation counsellors may use these theories to improve their practice. James Vargo examines cognitive approaches to counselling, and, although his chapter is concerned essentially with aspects of physical disabilities, and might be expected to be based within a health model of counselling, the general concerns and principles associated with it apply directly in other contexts. Importance of consumer identity, the issues of empowerment and choice are readily apparent within this context.

Thomas and Parker underline the importance of counsellors developing their own belief system, but recognize that this must be based on sound philosophical notions and an informed background in psychology. However, elsewhere other aspects are noted, including sociological views which relate disability to ecological climate and social perception. For example, Vargo examines the effects on the rehabilitation process, of the attitudes of the general public toward people with physical disabilities. Indeed, at one level it can be argued that disability is very much a feature of social patterns of thinking and experience. Using such a background, it becomes possible to see that disability, whether recognized under formal labels by health and educational services affects most individuals at some time in their lives. It is from this point of view that Holosko's chapter is a timely reminder of the effects that social conditions have on individuals who are not regarded as having a disability. Much of the impact is seen to be similar to that experienced by individuals with recognized disabilities. The issues relating to lack of empowerment, choice, regression of behaviour and inability to function effectively to overcome difficulties without external supports, including those of the family, are readily apparent. The interrelationship of these factors with recognized disabilities may make the situation much more devastating, thus the critical need to involve the process of rehabilitation counselling.

Both Thomas and Parker's and Brown's chapters recognize the importance of sound professional practice. It is recognized that professional practice must be based on sound theoretical constructs using clear applications of research to practice, even though practice must involve concerns over generalization. The sensitivity of counsellors and the way that they are educated are also seen as highly relevant issues, and many chapters underline the importance of moving to much more innovative practice in terms of education and training, with greater sensitivity towards the consumer, and much more involvement of the consumer in the selection of rehabilitation and counselling students, and in the evaluation of intervention effectiveness.

Particular practices which have not traditionally been featured as major rehabilitation strategies are raised in several chapters. Brown argues that the client's perception of his or her quality of life needs to be considered in designing any counselling intervention, while Webb notes that unfortunately, quality of life usually is not considered as a factor in rehabilitation. Probably one of the most important aspects of this relates to the goal of leisure time pursuits and the important role, in terms of psychological stability and development, that leisure plays in healthy performance or rehabilitation effectiveness. Day argues this has relevance to vocational re-employment and family adaptability, amongst other relevant characteristics. Holosko also talks about the importance of leisure time and leisure time planning.

Many of the critical features within this book relate to developmental models as evidenced in Robertson's chapter, which provides a general life transitions framework for counselling, with particular emphasis on adaptation to physical disabilities. Here and elsewhere the effects of regression during times of stress and loss are highlighted. This is well exemplified within Susan Webb's chapter, which examines grieving processes, and in Gary Hornby's chapter, which describes the process of adapting to a family member with a disability. Holosko notes that similar models have been developed to understand the reactions to becoming unemployed. Both Holosko and Robertson point out that many variables influence an individual's reaction to a transition event such as unemployment, and the counsellor needs to be mindful of these in rehabilitation counselling.

Several chapters focus on the relation of stress and coping as they pertain to the rehabilitation process. Both Kennett and Robertson emphasize the importance of assessing the client's coping strategies, encouraging use of those which are effective, and helping the client develop alternate methods of coping.

There are many points in the book where it is recognized that there are no functional differences, from a rehabilitation counselling point of view, in rehabilitation and habilitation. It is also recognized that there is no tangible end point that can be labelled as "rehabilitated" or "adjusted". Adaption, learning and rehabilitation are continuous processes which hopefully result in functional behaviour. Again, although there are accepted definitions of handicap and disability, these terms are sometimes used interchangeably. However, generally, the term "disability" refers to the basic physical or allied condition, while "handicap" refers to the environmental or psychological limitations imposed by the disability.

At this particular stage in the development of rehabilitation there appears to be increasing recognition of the role played by emotional factors on the one hand, and environmental factors on the other. The importance of qualitative evaluation and the recognition of introspective or internal factors to the individual in promoting change in development may come to be seen as some of the most important aspects of any healing or adaptive process. The recognition by Holosko that physiological factors are related to unemployment and manifest themselves in issues associated with stress and illness is similarly reflected in the chapter on grieving and loss associated with the writing of Susan Webb.

The personalized approach to stress by Backenroth from Sweden underlines the far-reaching change to a more personalized and psychological approach to various aspects of disability. Many of the points made by Backenroth are underlined by both Hornby and Webb and are also reflected in the chapters by Vargo and Robertson. Robertson and Backenroth also stress the importance of social environment and the networks developed within it in terms of impact on health and disability. Physical attributes of disease and poor functioning may be precipitated by inadequate components in the social network. Such views are far removed from the traditional medical approach of physical treatment. Obviously, both aspects of intervention are necessary, again stressing a view noted by both Brown and by Backenroth that control and choice are important in the hands of the consumer. Without this the consumers are unempowered and unable to develop the social networks which are so important in the minimization of handicap and in promoting effective health. Scientifically, there is a move away from purely quantitative results with a recognition that qualitative findings, though less easily calibrated and measured, almost by definition, play an important role in understanding the processes of disability.

Hornby, Robertson, Webb and Backenroth all stress the importance of family intervention and the perception of the person with the disability by members of the family. The importance of the Backenroth article is that it deals specifically with one population, namely people with deafness, yet the same types of findings recorded in her chapter are reflected in those written by authors concerned with other types of disability - mental handicap and physical disabilities. This again stresses the generality of many of the findings across disability domains.

It is extremely important to recognize that what may be appropriate for a medical model with specific intervention for particular physical disabilities may take a different form and require different procedures of scientific enquiry and application when considering social and psychological dimensions. Indeed, the isolation of professional personnel concerned with specific disabilities has, in the field of psychology and counselling, restricted the application of important knowledge across the domains of disability.

Backenroth as well as Brown, recognizes the importance of holistic approaches to counselling and rehabilitation. Backenroth stresses that many counsellors find they are engaged in psychotherapy and allied activities rather than vocational counselling. This underlines Brown's point that rehabilitation must be seen as broad ranging and reflect the needs and choices of the consumer, rather than as forcing individuals into previously arranged constructs derived from the needs of society, for example, the insistence of many advocates and vocational counsellors that people return rapidly to the workforce, regardless of whether there are more pressing problems and challenges.

There are other threads throughout the chapters. There is a clear recognition that although some aspects of counselling cover all groups with disabilities, there must also be a recognition that cultural differences require sensitivity amongst counsellors. Indeed, it is essential that counsellors receive professional education. An attempt should be made to include both cultural minorities and persons with disabilities themselves in the relevant professions. Further, in recent years, we have seen the evolution of language usage in reference to individuals with disabilities. It is no longer acceptable to use such words as disabled as an adjective describing the person (e.g., disabled person, deaf student) or as a noun describing a group of persons (e.g., the mentally handicapped). Such language can unintentionally conjure up stereotypical perceptions that mask a person's true characteristics and cause the user to see the individual as an object or disease. Counselling and rehabilitation are about people and the challenges over which those individuals request guidance or support. The currently acceptable terminology (e.g., people with disabilities, persons with deafness) serves to emphasize that disability is not a descriptor of the whole person but rather an attribute of the individual, as is eye colour (Humes, Szymanski and Hohenshil, 1989).

The implications of language can be taken further, for

Introduction

Holosko raises several points which are important in general terms. He shows that many of the factors affecting the general population in terms of unemployment produce and involve very similar symptoms confronting a wide range of people with disabilities. Thus, the disability/non-disability categories are unclear at the borders. There are generalities in arguments and practices in this area. Holosko also notes the complex interactions between variables, and the systemic nature of causation.

Although within one book it is not possible to cover all aspects of rehabilitation counselling, we have attempted to note major and common themes from different countries and in various aspects of disability. We also stress the importance of these rehabilitation skills being in the hands of all those who counsel as part of a professional delivery to consumers, who are encouraged to be responsible and controlling of their own rehabilitation process.

REFERENCES

Humes, C.W., Szymanski, E.M. and Hohenshil, T.H. (1989) 'Roles of counselling in enabling persons with disabilities', *Journal of Counselling and Development, 68,* 145-150.

Peavy, V., Robertson, S. and Westwood, M. (1982) 'Guidelines for Counsellor Education in Canada', *Canadian Counsellor, 16* (3), 135-143.

World Programme of Action Concerning Disabled Persons; 1983, United Nationals, New York.

Chapter Two

COMPETENCE ACQUISITION: THE ROLE OF THE PROFESSIONAL IN REHABILITATION

Hy I. Day

INTRODUCTION

> Language is the picture and counterpart of thought.
> Mark Hopkins, 1841

He just can't say goodbye
He just won't say goodbye
He just doesn't know how to say goodbye

Here are three statements, similar in form and, superficially, interchangeable. However, the connotations in these three statements are vastly different and reflect alternate approaches to an understanding of human behaviour. In fact, all we really know is that a person is complaining that someone is prolonging a conversation unduly. But each statement also carries implications about the cause of the conversation prolongation that reflect the listener's philosophy of human behaviour.

In the first statement the listener implies that the speaker is unable to terminate a conversation. In the second, the implication is that the speaker may have the ability but, of his own free will, chooses not to exercise it. The third statement implies that the speaker is unaware, or has not been taught the socially accepted manner of terminating a conversation.

Should the conversation prolonger ever come to a counsellor for assistance with the problem of undue prolongation of conversations, the counsellor must be aware of the approach he or she takes to identify the nature of the problem. The choice of intervention strategy will reflect the view of the counsellor in relation to his or her philosophy of human behaviour and the believed cause of the problems in social interaction terms. It should be noted the word "counsellor" is used as a generic name for the professional who is offering assistance to an individual, while recognizing that the word carries connotative meanings far beyond my intent.

The three statements are illustrative of three dominant models of human behaviour that guide the activities of counsellors in their daily work (Day, 1973). This chapter examines these models insofar as they are pertinent to an understanding of how counsellors interact with people with disabilities. Central to the discussion will be the concept of competence.

The chapter shows how the three models are reflected in the language and thought processes of a counsellor so that issues such as competence have different meanings and roles in practice. It is suggested that the counsellor must become cognizant of the models and the implications of their use since they shape all the counsellor/client interactions.

While the emphasis is on the rehabilitation of people with disabilities, it is impossible to compare the three models without extending the discussion to other situations and to the interaction of counsellors with people who do not have visible disabilities. The existence of disabilities is not restricted to people where they are apparent and obvious, and the nature of the counselling process is generalizable to a wide variety of situations.

Clear bias will be shown towards one of the models in the presentation because this author has a point of view and the chapter is designed to express it. But there is no attempt to denigrate any other model; each is appropriate in its place. The chapter is designed to alert the counsellor to the fact that all of these models exist and are in common use, and that they control the thought and language, as well as relationships, in the counselling act. When a counsellor becomes cognizant of the models that are influencing the interaction in a counselling situation, the counsellor will better understand the reasons for the client's reactions.

An architect's model of a building evokes an image of its final structure. However, models are never exact representations and embody distortions and relationships that are not found in reality. Similarly, the models presented here are not to be found as discrete entities in actual practice. Programmes and counsellors do not function exclusively within the constraints of a particular model. They shift back and forth among models depending on a large number of factors, not the least of which is the philosophy of the programme and of the individual. Readers may deny such shifts, but becoming aware of the phenomenon may help clarify relationships and enhance success in service delivery. Recognizing the dominant model being used may help explain why counselling sessions advance as they do.

Using language without recognition of the connotations in the words does not allow the counsellor to realize that the client may be using identical words in a different way. Language controls thought and thought controls relationships. We act differently with students than we do with clients, patients, or consumers. Students come to counsellors for different reasons than do consumers or patients.

The three models introduced in the three sentences at the beginning of this chapter will be examined under a number of headings. Table 2.1 presents a matrix of models by headings and gives an overly simplified representation of their relationships.

THE LEGAL/INDUSTRIAL MODEL

This model is ubiquitous in all aspects of our daily lives including social interaction and tends to guide our response to others. It is reflected in our everyday conventional language and in our expectations of the behaviour of ourselves and of others. The legal/industrial model carries with it a number of assumptions and beliefs.

Table 2.1 - Models of Human Behaviour

	LEGAL/INDUSTRIAL	MEDICAL	EDUCATIONAL
Motivational philosophy	Free-will	Determinism	Determinism
Goals	Ethical behaviour	Health, wellness	Competence
Organizational structure	Courts, workshops	Hospitals, clinics	Schools
Control	Conformity	Compliance	Obedience
Competence	Bestowed	Lost and regained	The goal
Rehabilitation	Self-directed control	Restoration of competence	Increasing competencies
Need for service	Inappropriate behaviour	Loss of competence	Low competence levels
Service provider	Police, employer	Medical & paramedical staff, counsellor	Teacher, instructor
Role of service provider	Advising, enforcing	Ministering, counselling	Teaching, instructing
Title of service recipient	Citizen, worker, consumer	Patient, client	Student

Motivational Philosophy

The model assumes that people have the ability to make free choices and, while influenced by their environments, are the final arbiters of their actions. The origin of the assumption lies somewhere in past history and is influenced by the philosophical question of "the purpose of human existence". Humans were envisioned to be created in the image of God and endowed with wisdom and insight somewhere between animals and angels. The nature of this wisdom allows them to discern between Good and Evil and therefore to make informed evaluations of their own behaviour.

Adults were expected to behave responsibly. Life was described as a struggle between the forces of Good and Evil and humans, because of their ability to make ethical judgments, were expected to choose actions that reflect judgements of goodness. In this way they were better than animals. But because their choices were not always morally correct, they were less than angels.

Responsibility for making ethically appropriate (socially acceptable) choices is entrusted to the individual. When a person acts in an inappropriate manner therefore, that person is the author of his or her own misfortune. This ability to select appropriate choices is termed competence.

Competence

Competence appears to be a characteristic of adulthood bestowed on people when they reach specific chronological ages. Such ages may be 16, in Ontario, Canada when people become competent to obey the laws of safe driving (but are not licensed to drive a vehicle unless they can demonstrate the required driving skills); 18, when people become competent to make a political decision and to run for political office; and 18, or 20, or 21, – depending on a governmental law - when they become competent to drink in public and to purchase liquor and cigarettes.

It should be emphasized that, in this meaning of the word, competence is the ability to make appropriate moral choices, not skill. One is viewed as competent to make decisions about driving behaviour, but must demonstrate driving skills and knowledge of regulations by passing an examination. Should the driver lose his or her licence to drive, it is assumed that the driver chose not to demonstrate skilful or knowledgeable behaviour and so permission is rescinded. At the same time there are laws that govern the behaviour of an unlicensed driver. That person is presumed to be competent, but has chosen to behave unethically, in driving without a licence.

Similarly a welder is awarded a certificate that attests to the fact that he or she has demonstrated an acceptable level of skill in welding. A job may be obtained on the basis of such a certificate. However, the worker may be fired from that job. Firing implies inadequate skills or lack of conformity to the rules of the workplace. For the latter instance it does not imply incompetence but rather wilful choice by the worker to act inappropriately on the job.

Children are not expected to be competent. The model suggests that children, like subhuman species of animals, are motivated by instincts and are not rational. They are not expected to be able to distinguish Good from Evil, or to choose freely to behave ethically, and the reaction of our courts to crimes committed by children reflects this.

However, some adults never have competence bestowed on them. We call these "incompetent" adults "mentally handicapped" or "developmentally delayed" and treat them as we do children. We do not expect competent behaviour from them and when they act in a rational manner we may become confused and unwilling to accept their behaviour as if it were that of a competent person.

Rehabilitation

While not alien to rehabilitation, the Legal/Industrial Model does not concern itself with change. Rather, its primary concern is the maintenance of existing behaviour. This is accomplished by developing sets of rules and regulations and enforcing conformity.

It is expected that members of the society, cultural, or

employment group will work to maintain those skills that will keep them within the mainstream of the society. Societies are not static but change in attitude and in the demands made on their members. Members are expected to adjust to the changes in order to maintain their status within the group. Members are expected to choose to conform to those behaviour patterns deemed ethical within the definition of the society.

Where change in behaviour patterns towards conformity is required, the model does not supply the wherewithal to change, but expects that members will use such facilities and methodologies that are available to them to adjust. These methodologies are inherent in the other two models that will be presented later.

Rehabilitation programmes frequently run workshops which are simulated industrial or clerical settings whose goals are to improve vocational aptitude and skills. The workshops themselves, however, are not designed to induce change; they simply provide a milieu for change to take place and the conditions for practicing new skills. Direction is provided by counsellors and instructors who use techniques based on other models to effect appropriate changes. Thus, while a vocational rehabilitation centre is in part an industrial concern, the activities within it are shaped by the models that dominate.

Trainees are expected to make socially acceptable choices within the levels of skill they have achieved. They are rewarded for conformity as expected by the Industrial model and for skill attainment as expected in an Educational model by promotions and financial reward.

Advocacy and peer groups tend to accept this model and maintain that their members are competent, have the right to make free decisions and should be treated by society as are other competent members.

Example:
>A car driver exceeds the speed limit on the highway and is pulled over by a police officer.
>"Are you aware that you are exceeding the speed limit?" "Do you have a licence to drive?" "I must give you a citation for driving too fast!"

Implied in these statements is the belief that the driver

has demonstrated a sufficiently high level of skills to have been awarded a licence to drive, but has abused the award wilfully by driving at excessive speed. Non-conformity elicits punishment imposed by the police officer who represents society's values as interpreted through its laws.

Behind all of this is the implication that conformity is satisfying and people should prefer to choose obedience to authority. Thus punishment is justified because "it's for your own good" and we should take the punishment to heart and obey rules and regulations.

Nature of Control

According to the Legal/Industrial model, society defines morality and individuals are expected to conform. Choice to conform is, of course, wilful and society expects it. Reward is seldom extended by society to people who conform, although highly skilful behaviour is maintained by promotions, wage raises, election and the conferring of certificates, degrees and titles. On the other hand, failure to conform, as well as inept behaviour, is punished by demotion and discharge, by fines, incarcerations, and confiscation of certification. Thus we find that punishment is the normal method of establishing and maintaining conformity in people, whether competent or incompetent, whether skilful or unskilful.

Conformity is maintained by the use of judges, employers, unions, or clubs and other social organizations. Conformity is also maintained by making people who do not conform feel guilty and inadequate. This is extended by advertisers into many domains, so that people choose the appropriate deodorants, foods, sex objects and burial plots. People who conform are called citizens, employees, and consumers.

Role of the Service Provider

When the speeders come to an authority figure, they are coming for reprimand and/or advice. They may choose to accept or reject the expected behaviour patterns that are spelled out to them. Sometimes rejection of the service may keep an unrepentant advisee incarcerated or unemployed. Sometimes the advisee may seek other advice from more sympathetic advisers.

Such advisers are lawyers, judges, and police in legal instances and employers, peers, and vocational or placement officers in employment instances. In social situations where the individual seeks help in making a decision, advice may be solicited from anyone, family, friends, even radio phone-in hosts. In economic situations financial consultants may be sought. But the final choice is always that of the individual and is made within available constraints.

Sometimes rehabilitation counsellors are called on to act as advisors. The individual (member of society) may come to the counsellor to inquire where and how to arrange for services such as housing, finances, or employment. At such times the professional must distinguish between acting as an advisor and giving advice, as a case coordinator and recommending service, or as a counsellor and giving counsel. Counselling, in this case, is more than merely information or opinion. It is giving guidance or leadership to one who is unable to decide alone.

But rarely do counsellors assume the Legal/Industrial model in their professional work. Out of their offices they may adopt the model in interaction with colleagues, spouses, shopkeepers, and friends. But not with consumers. Rehabilitation counsellors do not, as a rule, call them "consumers". Rather they tend to call them "clients", and treat them as persons in distress who require guidance in the form of expert, professional assistance to overcome their distress. But are these clients in distress or ill? Or are we confusing disability with distress and viewing these clients as ill?

People with obvious disabilities may be ill. But people without obvious disabilities may also be ill. People with disabilities may be distressed and require professional assistance to alleviate their distress. But they may also require advice and guidance to make appropriate choices.

THE CLINICAL/MEDICAL MODEL

A man has committed a crime and killed an innocent victim. The full weight of the Legal/Industrial system has been brought to bear. He has been arrested, given access to a lawyer, a judge and a court, and the prosecutor, following the accepted system, argues that the individual has wilfully committed a crime, breaking the laws of society. Punishment is therefore sought by the prosecuting lawyer. But the defense lawyer shifts from the Legal/Industrial model to a Clinical/Medical model of human behaviour. The defense lawyer calls a clinician or medical practitioner to the stand, who argues that the accused was not competent at the moment the crime was committed.

Example:
> Defense Lawyer - "Was the accused acting wilfully when he committed the crime?"
> Expert, clinical witness - "No, the man was acting on an irresistible urge. At the time of the murder, he was acting with diminished capacity. He was not competent to appreciate his behaviour."

The model within which the expert, clinical witness is working believes that there are urges or impulses over which a person has no control and that competence can be diminished. The Clinical/Medical model is thus based on a number of such premises and it is important that these are compared with those of the Legal/Industrial model.

Motivational Philosophy

Following biological science, behaviour of humans, like that of subhuman species of animals, is seen to follow the principle of *determinism*. Behaviour is orderly and potentially predictable. People are not free to choose their behaviour because it is determined by external or internal, biological forces.

Rehabilitation

Rehabilitation, in the language of the Medical model, is defined as "the ultimate restoration of a disabled person to his maximum capacity - physical, emotional, and vocational" (Rusk and Hilleboe, 1965). It is a form of medical therapy and is mainly concerned with the loss and restoration of physical function. Itoh and Lee (1982) argue that rehabilitation should be initiated at the earliest possible time, in fact as soon as the diagnosis is established, and should be considered an integral part of what they call secondary prevention.

This follows from the approach that rehabilitation for clients/patients is based on the assumption that competence can be lost and restored. The client/patient is re-habilitated to the previously healthy state or as close to it as possible.

Medical rehabilitation deals mainly with the loss and restoration of physical or mental function. It utilizes medical and paramedical personnel who minister to the patient and restore him or her to the healthiest condition possible. This restoration or rehabilitation process requires that the patient adopt a compliant role in which he or she is the recipient of treatment and follows the directions and orders given by the professional staff. Rehabilitation is perceived as the final stages of therapy.

Competence

Competence is equated with health and people lose competence following an event such as a ski accident, or through a disease, stress, or the aging process. Competence is generally lost in one or more domains but can be maintained in others. People who suffer the loss of physical competence are assumed to have retained mental competence but it is recognized that a traumatic event may result in loss of competence to make appropriate decisions.

The person who has committed a murder is deemed to have lost mental competence either temporarily (temporary insanity) or permanently. The court may therefore hand over jurisdiction of the prisoner, who now becomes a patient, to the authorities of the Clinical/Medical model for incarceration in an institute modelled on Clinical/Medical principles.

Within the Medical model, mental illness is generally considered to be the result of a biological dysfunction or the outcome of a traumatic event that occurred to the individual and resulted in that person's loss of mental competence. In this case the individual is seen to be unable (incompetent) to make appropriate decisions and so these must be made by others - psychiatrists, counsellors, or family.

Clinical psychiatry is concerned with the loss and restoration of mental or psychological competence. The process of restoration, like that in physical medicine, is seen to proceed through a number of stages, the final one termed rehabilitation. Thus psychiatric rehabilitation is viewed as a natural step of service delivery within the confines of a psychiatric hospital, a psychiatric ward of a general hospital, or a clinic, which often serves as the bridge between inpatient therapeutic service and continued post-discharge service.

Moreover, one consequence of mental incompetence is seen as the impairment of physical and social competence and, in such cases patients do not care for their health needs, feed themselves, or socialize appropriately. Most hospitals recognize this and offer rehabilitative care to compensate for these losses. This may lead to the dispute of whether the restoration of mental competence would also restore other competencies or whether counselling is required as a separate and distinct addition.

In some medical institutions the Legal/Industrial model has intruded and deems the patients to be adults and entitled to grieve inequities, to choose therapies, and vote in elections. Clearly these are intrusions with the implication that the patients have not lost their capacities (competence) to choose and make decisions.

The word *rehabilitation* reflects the Clinical/Medical model. It connotes the restoration to a previous state of health or capacity (competence) and requires the acceptance of the notion that previous competence existed. While this may be true with physical disablement, it is difficult to rationalize when dealing with cognitive or emotional competence. It is especially true when dealing with an individual who has reached the socially determined chronological ages of competence but has failed to display anticipated modes of behaviour. Clearly one could not label an intervention as restorative when competence had never been gained and lost, and so the term *habilitation* has been introduced.

Control

Where the Legal/Industrial model demands conformity to an authority, the Clinical/Medical model requires compliance to the authority; compliance in taking medication, exercising, stopping drinking or smoking, and compliance in thought process. Insight, the goal of some psychotherapies, is the acknowledgement by a patient of the appropriateness of the therapist's interpretation of the problem and so is really a measure of the patient's compliance to the norms of the therapist. Behavioural therapies require that the instrumental behaviour of the client/patient comply with the expectations of the therapist.

Without compliance, the counsellor or therapist cannot control the counselling situation. Control is manifested in a large number of ways: choosing the time and place of meetings, controlling the language style and content, and having a large array of rewards and punishments. Since the client/patient is coming for help while in distress, the counsellor has at his or her disposal the ability to minister to, or withhold succour to, the client/patient. Although the goal of rehabilitation is supposed to be independence, the counsellor must wrestle with the problem of how to bestow independence in an environment of dependency.

Role of Service Provider

In the Medical/Clinical model the service provider is a medical, a medical surrogate, or a paramedical, staff person. Training may be in any of the health-allied fields including clinical psychology. The staff person is usually designated as a clinician, therapist or counsellor.

The style of interaction used by the therapist/counsellor is determined by the job description, the training of the individual, and his or her method of communication. Occupational therapists, for example, may be trained to assess and improve the physical competencies of the patient. To this end, the therapist will prepare a set of scales or other types of measures and a set of activities likely to influence competencies in those areas of concern. Actually, the role of the occupational therapist is

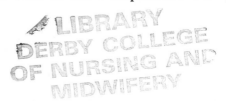
21

probably more like that of a teacher since the activity is that of changing levels of competence (see the next section of this chapter for detail).

Rehabilitation counsellors, when working within the Medical/Clinical model, do not act as advisors, but as experts who help patients/clients become aware of their feelings, attitudes, and actions. The way they approach this task reflects their personal beliefs and *modus operandi*. They are interested in modifying pathologies, and personality or cognitive styles. They believe that behaviour is symptomatic of underlying physical, emotional, or mental dysfunction. But frequently they depart from application of the Medical/Clinical model to that of the Education model which will be examined next. It would therefore be appropriate to reserve discussions of the role of the counsellor until later.

Rehabilitation then, in the Clinical/Medical model, is the restoration of competence to an individual. There is a wide array of instruments and tests that are used to measure competent behaviour so that loss can be identified in kind and degree. While the Clinical/Medical model tends to be identified as a qualitative one in which people are seen to be healthy or ill, this view is oversimplistic. Medical and paramedical wisdom has certainly become quantity referenced so that change in heart rate can be monitored, and IQ score deviation from "normal" can be measured. Degree of diminished capacity can be evaluated, and Rorschach and TAT responses can be given numerical values on various dimensions. The restoration of competence can be complete or incomplete so that the patient may be left with 70% of previous gait or greater than previous level of smoking control. But this quantification of competence is a result of the contamination of the pure Clinical/Medical model by the next model we have to examine.

THE EDUCATIONAL MODEL

One day, on a phone-in programme on the radio, the topic for discussion was homosexuality and the rights of gay and homosexual persons to work in educational systems. Telephone callers seemed to represent two distinct groups.

In the first group were those who believed that

homosexuality was biological or physiological and that people couldn't help themselves. Included in this group were those who suggested that homosexuals were sick and that there was no known cure. On the other hand the group also included homosexual people who phoned in and told how it came to them as a revelation that they were sexually different.

Example:
> "I woke up one morning at the age of twelve and
> just knew that I was gay."

Depending on whether they considered homosexuality to be a disease or a lifestyle these callers displayed pity or pride. But none of them argued that homosexual teachers should be kept out of classrooms.

In the second group were callers who insisted that homosexual teachers should not be allowed in classrooms. Their fear was not that children would be contaminated, but that the children might learn to like the "way of life" of the homosexual teacher and adopt it.

These latter callers viewed homosexuality within an Educational model and assumed that the etiology of homosexuality lay in reinforced behaviour initiated through social learning or imitation. If their children were to remain heterosexual, homosexuals would have to be segregated and devalued so they could not serve as role models.

The Educational model is much more ubiquitous than we realize and affects our attitudes towards, and interactions with, other people, including children. The model is based on the assumption that all instrumental acts can be learned under conditions of reinforcement and punishment. But of the two the Educational model puts greater emphasis on reinforcement. Skinner, in fact, in his book *Walden Two* (1945), makes the point that punishment is inadequate to change behaviour permanently and that positive reinforcement produces permanent behaviour change.

Motivational Philosophy

The educational model rejects the notion of free-will in favour of determinism and potential predictability of behaviour. Control is an important goal in science and requires that one accepts the philosophy that behaviour is determined and that the motivations to act are identifiable and can be manipulated.

Competence

Greif and Matarazzo (1982) define rehabilitation as "the learning process by which a person who has suffered physical, intellectual, and/or personality changes (secondary to injury or disease) recovers functioning to the extent possible, develops compensatory skills in areas where deficits persist, and adjusts emotionally to the level of functioning attained" (p.3).

Comparison of this definition to that of Rusk and Hilleboe (1965) highlights the subtle, but important, differences in philosophy. The latter puts emphasis on "restoration" compared with "recovers functioning" (a more active verb) and Greif and Matarazzo's definition includes "develops compensatory skills", a clear reference to developing competence under the circumstances of the changes brought about by injury or disease.

Similarly Trieschmann (1988), in practical terms, defined rehabilitation as "teaching people to live with their disability in their own environment" (p.26). Learning is a dynamic process. Such learning begins when the injury occurs and goes on throughout the individual's life. "There is no tangible endpoint that can be labelled as 'rehabilitated' or 'adjusted' because people with disabilities are continually learning to adapt to their environment in, hopefully, more functional and satisfying ways" (p.26). This statement is an even clearer exposition of the Educational model's approach to competence. It should be noted that none of the definitions have dealt with congenital or prenatal conditions that make habilitation necessary. Frequently these are conditions that are limiting to intellectual, physical, and emotional growth in childhood and fit into the rubric of "special education". But when the individual reaches the age of chronological maturity, he or she is transferred to some type of "rehabilitation" service that delivers continuing education.

Anthony (Anthony and Jansen, 1984) distinguishes

between "recidivism" and "rehabilitation". He suggests that the concern of the former is with health-illness problems and is related to diagnostic determinants. The latter, on the other hand, is concerned with function and, in his outline of "psychosocial rehabilitation" (Anthony, 1979), the analysis of activities that will return rewards to the individual. There is little interest in diagnostics and symptomatology and more on skills and competence.

Since the Educational model is so concerned with the achievement of competence, the concept of competence needs to be defined in this context. Robert W. White (1959) was perhaps the first psychologist to describe scientifically the concept of competence. He defined it as "an organism's capacity to interact effectively with its environment" (p. 297). In this seminal paper he reviewed the literature to that time showing that competence is an inherent motivator in all organisms that leads them to increase the satisfaction that can be obtained from interaction with the environment. He noted Freud's (actually Hendrick's [1942] interpretation of Freudian theory) proposal of an instinct of mastery of the environment and its importance in developing an ego. He referred to Hebb's argument that people need to raise their levels of stimulation, Leuba's concept of optimal stimulation, and Berlyne's theory of exploratory behaviour. He defined competence according to Webster's dictionary as fitness or ability and noted the synonyms of capability, capacity, efficiency, proficiency, and skill. Finally he named the motivation that drives the need for competence – effectance.

Clearly White, and those that followed and developed his formulations (Connolly and Bruner, 1974), assumed that there is an intrinsic motivation to maximize satisfaction. But they failed to include one part of the definition of competence – effort required to achieve satisfaction. Competence *then* is better defined as:

> The maximization of satisfaction and the minimization of dissatisfaction with least effort. The ultimately competent person would therefore be able to act in such a way as to obtain maximum satisfaction in no time at all.

Clearly an ideal and one that cannot be attained. Thus we must accept the notion that, looking at behaviour through the Educational model, humans are at various stages of competence. But at the same time we recognize that competence is a quantifiable variable and that we are able to measure it.

> Johnny is a boy in Grade 6 spending much of his time in school, an institution which applies the Educational model. His teacher gives him a set of examinations to measure how far Johnny has reached on the competence continuum. In a series of 20 minute tests Johnny achieves the following scores: 75 in English Literature, 40 in Art, 100 in Geography, and 100 in Mathematics, having completed the last test in 15 minutes rather than the allotted 20 minutes. From this we conclude that Johnny is not very competent in Art and highly competent in Mathematics; even more highly competent than in Geography, as demonstrated by the speed with which he completed his test.

But suppose the teacher had given Johnny the Grade 8 Mathematics test. Chances are that he would do poorly on it, for he had never learned the material and so should not be expected to demonstrate competency in it.

Clearly, one must recognize the existence of many competencies and realize that their levels are functions of the time and place, the domain or area of expertise and the criterion groups that serve for comparison. Johnny may be more competent than other pupils in some domains in the sixth grade. At home he may be much less competent than his twin brother in making his bed, whittling, playing piano, and carrying out the garbage.

A study was conducted in a psychiatric hospital that illustrates this point. The hospital was in the midwestern United States and, as with so many psychiatric institutions on the edge of town, had large, lush grounds and so patients with ground privileges were able to take advantage of these.

Once a month each patient was normally brought to a staff meeting at which his or her status was updated and notes were written into the file. The patient participated at the meeting, but as a patient, not as a member of the group.

In the study, half of the subjects, who were all patients with ground privileges, were told, on the way to the staff meeting, that the focus of the meeting was to determine if ground privileges were to be denied. The other half of the subjects were told that the meeting might result in their discharge from the hospital. Behaviour of the patients at the meeting was gauged by the staff which was unaware of the study.

The results showed that the patients who were threatened with loss of ground privileges behaved in a sane and mentally competent manner. The patients threatened with discharge, on the other hand, behaved inappropriately. The researchers concluded that the patients were highly satisfied with the quality of their lives and knew how to maximize their satisfaction.

Clearly the patients in the hospital were fairly competent in manipulating their environment. But one could not extrapolate from this that they would be equally competent living in the community. Rehabilitation, for them, was not necessary to continue their stay in the hospital. In fact, there was no purpose in effecting change since the patients were not dissatisfied with their current conditions.

Rehabilitation

Rehabilitation can be defined as the process of teaching an individual the skills or competencies required to maximize satisfactions with minimum effort within the community in which the individual is expected to live. In fact, this definition is no different than the one used in education, and rehabilitation could be renamed Special Education or Re-education. Moreover, the characteristics of the Educational model can be transposed directly and the roles of the participants in the process can be viewed as those of Adult Education.

The goals and objectives of the educational system are to accept students into programmes at lower levels of competencies and graduate them at higher levels. The methods may vary from one institution to another, but the goals and objectives are identical.

The curriculum in rehabilitation may differ from that of a

university or trade school, but a number of characteristics are common:

1.   There is a curriculum of subjects available at the training centre. The student selects those courses he or she deems appropriate, usually with guidance from members of the staff.
2.   The entry level to a subject is measured on a quantitative metre. To gain entry, the student must demonstrate a level of competence appropriate to the entry criterion for the subject.
3.   Each course has a fixed length of time and its goals and objectives are clarified to the student at a point when the student can still make a realistic determination of the appropriateness of enrolment.
4.   At specified times during the course, the student is evaluated and receives feedback so that adjustment in the work style of the student, or the course contents or teaching strategies can be made.
5.   Upon completion of the term a final evaluation is conducted and the degree of progress is determined. If the student has reached a predetermined criterion of acceptable competence for that course, a report of successful completion is issued. In the event that the criterion has not been reached, a reappraisal is made and a determination is made on whether the course should be repeated.
6.   With successful completion of a course decisions are made as to the appropriateness of enrolling in another course or courses, graduation from the programme, or terminating the educational programme.

Role of service provider

The professional, in this model, is neither a counsellor, a police officer, nor a supervisor. Rather, the professional who is offering help and guidance adopts the role of a teacher or instructor.

The teacher's function is to raise competencies to a level where the student will improve his or her coping skills and hence quality of life, by having greater control over those areas which do not allow the maximization of satisfaction with minimum effort. The teacher must act as any adult educational system would expect: identify the competencies that are required in order to allow the student to integrate maximally into society; measure the base levels of these competencies; apply educational principles to improve competencies in those areas in which the teacher is him or herself competent; and evaluate the student's progress through the educational enterprise.

As a counsellor, the professional might not be willing to separate the various areas of the client's life, having been trained to believe that all of them are so intertwined that affecting one affects all. Moreover, the counsellor is taught to assume that effective change can be accomplished by the same person in many domains of life.

But teachers in adult education tend to be specialists. The teacher may have specialized in vocational skills training, social skills training, or life skills training, or a combination of these skills. The number of skills is great and the levels of skills to which the training programmes extend are many. The teacher is not compelled to be an expert in all the areas.

As a poor, struggling graduate student, this writer undertook to teach an Introductory Psychology course in the extension department of his university. While clearly not an expert in the field, I felt sufficiently competent to instruct adults who were coming to take a non-degree course in the area I was trying to master. But what became clear in the first evening was the high level of competence that existed in areas other than psychology among the Introductory Psychology students. Economically, most members of the class were obviously more successful than the instructor. Socially, many had graces that were superior to mine. But they had come to learn in the narrow domain of psychological wisdom. They did not want to be taught things beyond the curriculum, although it must be admitted that some of them had a much broader definition of psychology and its utility than I had.

The role of the teacher is to teach skills. Fortunately, the teacher is helped by the existence of the intrinsic motivation of effectance. The teacher who recognizes that this innate motivation is always present, also recognizes that the student does not need to be motivated, but directed.

A frequent complaint of teachers is that their students aren't motivated. These children usually do not have their curricula adjusted or the style of teaching altered. Rather, the Medical model intrudes and they are sent to a psychologist or social worker for testing and therapy. They diagnose the children to find the underlying reasons for non-compliance with the goals of the teacher. The Medical model leads these professionals to regard "poor motivation" as a symptom of an underlying illness rather than as a conflict of motives.

But motivation, as outlined by Hebb (1955), has two components - level and direction. Level of motivation tends to be a function of health, and it must be assumed that all healthy people (with or without disabilities) have a fairly high level of motivation.

> Assuming the individual is healthy (although he or she may have a disability), the problem then is really one of direction. When the teacher complains about lack of motivation, it is actually a complaint about obedience. The teacher wants the student to be motivated to achieve the goals that the teacher has deemed to be important to the student. This may result in a conflict between the teacher who is directing the student one way and the student to whom these goals are of secondary importance. The student resists and appears to be disobedient or lazy. The student, however, is resisting the demands of accepting the goals of the teacher.

Similarly, students in rehabilitation training are motivated. But they may be motivated to protect those levels of competence that they already have. Moving from one situation to another means becoming less competent in the new situation, with accompanying feelings of doubt, fear and anxiety just like the situation where Johnny, in Grade 6, was given the Grade 8 mathematics test. It seems far safer to them not to change than to abandon their present situation. This is especially true for those who have suffered a traumatic experience or who have rarely tasted the success of achieving higher levels of competencies. Rather than label these persons as lazy, unmotivated, or malingerers, the professional must recognize the underlying motives that restrict the learner's willingness to change.

The recognition that motivation must be redirected rather than increased, forces the instructor to become cognizant of those conditions that alter behaviour. Students may fear the unknown because it appears more threatening than the present conditions which, though seemingly uncomfortable, may be the best to which the student aspires. There may be fear of losing competence when moving into new conditions and this fear may be exacerbated by previous failures. Teachers must recognize these trepidations and focus their efforts in easing the student through the transition from higher competence at low level of achievement to temporarily reduced competence that will eventually result in a higher level of reward in interaction with the environment. They must create opportunities in which students will succeed and so become more willing to attempt new and difficult transitions.

FINAL WORDS

Having outlined three models of human behaviour it does not follow that any single one should be adopted and applied to the exclusion of the others. It would be impossible to think and conduct one's interactions, including those in a job, while locked into one model. Rather, it is important to recognize that all three models exist in parallel and affect one's thoughts and actions.

At times the rehabilitation worker is called upon to act within the Legal/Industrial model and give someone friendly advice. To share one's thoughts and feelings as an equal, giving advice that can be rejected without rancour. There are times that one must counsel. One must help the client achieve a new definition of self, and a better understanding of how the client is coping with exigencies in life. But most of all the rehabilitation worker must be a teacher and assist in the development of competencies. The teacher must introduce concepts of learning and motivation to enhance the programme of skill development. Habeck and Fuller (1985) discuss this fully in a paper in which they advocate a "psychoeducational" perspective, one in which psychological contributions to the educational model are emphasized.

The ordinary student is motivated by effectance; the motive that White argued drives the need for competence. Students with a history of repeated failure may have created blocks to withstand change. Change can be fearful if it leads to uncertainly (Day and Berlyne, 1971). Better to remain locked in the present situation which may not be as optimally satisfying, but will have to do, than to venture into situations where one would feel even less competent. At such times all three models must be utilized, one must be a friend, a counsellor, and a teacher.

But when the counsellor switches back and forth among the models without letting the client know clearly which model is being applied at that moment, or even knowing him or herself which one is being practised, confusion in communications is sure to arise. Awareness of the existence of the models and their effect on the relationship is essential. Counsellors must be cognizant of the times and places for each, and communicate their selection to the client.

Depending on the educational background of the rehabilitation worker, one model may be preferred over the others. But the primary model should be educational with the other models adopted only when appropriate. And the counsellor must call on these models knowingly, and communicate shifts in models clearly.

REFERENCES

Anthony, W.A. (1979) *The Principles of Psychiatric Rehabilitation*, University Park Press, Baltimore.

Anthony, W.A. and Jansen, M.A. (1984) 'Predicting the Vocational Capacity of the Chronically Mentally Ill: Research and Policy Implications', *American Psychology, 39*, 537–544.

Connolly, K. and Bruner, J. (1974) *The Growth of Competence*, Academic Press, London.

Day, H.I. (1973) 'Models, Magic and Vocational Ministration', *Comeback, 1(3)*, 7–13.

Day, H.I. and Berlyne, D.I. (1971) 'Intrinsic Motivation', in G. Lesser (ed) *Psychology and Educational Practice*, Scott Foresman, Chicago, 294-335.

Greif, E. and Matarazzo, R.G. (1982) *Behavioral Approaches to Rehabilitation*, Springer Publishing Co. Inc., New York.

Habeck, R.V. and Fuller, T.C. (1985) 'Rehabilitation Counselling: A Psychoeducational Perspective', *Journal of Applied Rehabilitation Counselling*, 16, 43-47.

Hebb, D.O. (1955) 'Drives and the CNS (Conceptual Nervous System)', *Psychological Review*, 62, 243-354.

Hendrick, I. (1942) 'Instinct and the Ego During Infancy', *Psychoanalytical Quarterly*, 11, 33-58.

Hopkins, Mark (1841) 'An Address Delivered at the Dedication of Williston Seminary, East Hampton, Massachusetts', quoted in *The Home Book of Quotations*, December 1.

Itoh, M. and Lee, M.H.M. (1982) 'The Epidemiology of Disability as Related to Rehabilitation Medicine', in F.J. Kottke, G.K. Stillwell, and J.F. Lehmann (eds), *Krusen's Handbook of Physical Medicine and Rehabilitation* , Saunders: Philadelphia, (3rd ed).

Rusk, H.A. and Hilleboe, H.E. (1965) 'Rehabilitation', in H.E. Hilleboe, and G.W. Larimore (eds), *Preventative Medicine*, W.B. Saunders, Philadelphia.

Skinner, B.F. (1945) *Walden Two*, MacMillan, New York.

Trieschmann, R.B. (1988) *Spinal Cord Injuries: Psychological, Social and Vocational Rehabilitation* (2nd ed), Demos Publications, New York.

White, R.W. (1959) 'Motivation Reconsidered: The Concept of Competence', *Psychological Review*, 66, 297-333.

Chapter Three

APPLICATIONS OF THEORY TO REHABILITATION COUNSELLING PRACTICE

Kenneth R. Thomas and Randall M. Parker

INTRODUCTION

Students frequently comment that the theories presented in the courses they take are irrelevant to rehabilitation counselling practice. It is almost as though theory and practice were somehow divorced from each other and unrelated. Another possibility is that often persons interested in practice are simply not interested in research and theory. They are people-oriented as opposed to being data-oriented.

As rehabilitation counsellor educators, we cannot imagine a counselling practice which is not based on theory. Even the act of being nice to people is based on a conception of why being nice to people is "good for them". The same is true for activities which are not so nice, such as aloofness or punishment. The existence of theory is what makes a profession a profession. It provides a rationale for clinical interventions and a basis for prediction. In the words of Kurt Lewin, "There is nothing so practical as a good theory" (Lewin, 1951, p. 169).

WHY IS THEORY NECESSARY AND USEFUL?

Theory in rehabilitation counselling would be absolutely unnecessary if everything about rehabilitation clients, the rehabilitation counselling process, and society-at-large were known. In effect, there would be one theory, the "right"[1] one. Such, however, is not the case. There is much about the nature of counselling, disability, and career development that is not known. The "right" theory depends too much on the perspective of the observer. What is "right" for the behaviourist may never be right for the psychodynamic or person-centred counsellor. In view of this situation, it is necessary for the practitioner to rely on theory, ideally a theory or combination of theories which is congruent with his or her own perspective and offers potential to explain, predict, and ameliorate the client's behaviour.

Theory is useful because it allows the practitioner to choose "reasonable" and consistent intervention strategies. For example, if a practitioner is operating from a person-centred frame of reference, the offering of the "core conditions" makes sense in terms of facilitating self-exploration and decision-making. Similarly, counsellors utilizing Holland's occupational typology theory will seek to promote congruence between the client's personality type and the work environment because they believe that this is the surest way to promote job satisfaction and job satisfactoriness. It is critically important, therefore, that counselling students become familiar with theory, because without theory the profession would be stagnant, and practitioners could do little more than flounder in the dark.

CRITERIA FOR EVALUATING THEORIES

Corsini (1981) has identified 150 different approaches to counselling and psychotherapy. In addition, there are about a dozen major approaches to explaining occupational choice and career development (Brown, et al., 1984; Osipow, 1983). To even the most gifted rehabilitation counsellor or educator, this is an imposing number of theoretical offerings, especially since few of these theories were developed with disability and rehabilitation specifically in mind. The question becomes not only which of these theories is right for the practitioner, but also which will

---

[1] Portions of this chapter were adapted from material previously published in Thomas, K.R., Butler, A.J. and Parker, R.M. (1987) 'Psychosocial Counselling', in R.M. Parker (ed) *Rehabilitation Counselling: Basics and Beyond*, Pro-Ed, Austin, TX.

explain behaviour and thus offer clues for assisting rehabilitation clients.

Thomas, Butler and Parker (1987) have presented a systematic model for evaluating the appropriateness of specific theoretical approaches to counselling in a rehabilitation context. A modified version of this model is presented below to assist students and practitioners to evaluate theories of counselling, occupational choice, and career development.

One of the most important criteria in evaluating a theory is whether the philosophical notions underlying the theory are congruent with the counsellor's own belief system. For example, it is unlikely that a counsellor who valued highly the necessity of strong societal impositions to tame the innately savage nature of humans would feel very comfortable with an approach to counselling which emphasized the creation of a permissive counselling climate, such as that advocated by the person-centred theorists. A similar problem confronts the counsellor who places a premium on individuality and yet treats clients as if they absolutely must fit into one of the six personality types in Holland's career typology. The point is that theories of personal and career behaviour almost always embody assumptions about the relative influence of biological, social, and personal factors in shaping human development and behaviour, and it behooves the counsellor to make certain that these assumptions are in reasonable accord with his or her own beliefs and experience.

Another important criterion for evaluating theories is whether the theory is well-developed and generalizable to a wide range of human problems and concerns. Examples of particularly well-developed theories are those of Sigmund Freud, Carl Rogers, B.F. Skinner, Donald Super, John Holland, and E.G. Williamson. A related concern is how well verified the theoretical bases of the theory are and what, if any, empirical evidence is available to support the theory. Many theories in counselling and career choice offer little in the way of empirical evidence to support their claims of explanation and prediction (e.g., reality therapy, Adlerian therapy, Jungian analysis, Gestalt therapy, Ginzberg *et al.*'s theory (1951), and McMahon's Model of Vocational Redevelopment), whereas others offer considerable, if not compelling, evidence in support of their perspective (e.g., psychoanalysis, behavioural counselling, person-centred counselling, Holland's career typology, Super's developmental self-concept theory, and the Minnesota Theory of Work Adjustment). If counsellors are more than modern-day shamans, they should utilize strategies and techniques which are supported by research for use with relevant groups of clients and problem situations.

Another consideration is the range and type of client who can feasibly be served by an approach. Almost all of the approaches to counselling place some limitations on the range of clients which can be effectively served. For example, it is only in recent years that any credence at all was given to treating severely emotionally disturbed clients using psychoanalytic techniques. Moreover, it is debatable whether persons with limited cognitive abilities can benefit from any of the verbal therapies with the possible exception of behaviour modification and/or simple, repetitive cognitive interventions. (It should, however, be pointed out that we believe that virtually all clients will respond to a caring, warm, and empathic counselling climate.) In other words, are there limits imposed on the approach by such factors as the client's presenting problems, intellectual functioning, verbal expressivity, or counselling expectations?

Another criterion is what demands the approach makes on the counsellor with respect to training, experience, personality attributes, verbal ability, and values. Counselling approaches vary widely in their requirements for training and in terms of other demands that they make on the counsellor. For example, in the United States, psychoanalytic counselling, Adlerian therapy, Gestalt therapy, rational-emotive therapy, and reality therapy require post-graduate training in privately-run institutes which have been established to teach skills in applying specific techniques. Other approaches (e.g., trait-and-factor counselling, person-centred counselling, and behavioural counselling) are often taught as part of the counsellor's regular academic training. If a counsellor is going to utilize a particular approach, it is imperative that adequate training has been received. Similarly, the approach selected should be congruent with the counsellor's own personality attributes. For example, it is doubtful that talkative, cognitively-oriented, opinionated counsellors would be particularly effective or satisfied person-centred counsellors, but they might be very effective rational-emotive therapists.

Whether the goals of the counselling approach are congruent with the goals of the agency/facility in which the counsellor is employed is another important factor. In rehabilitation settings, the goals are often very specific and time-limited. Some approaches (e.g., the trait-and-factor and behavioural approaches) are better suited for specific, time-limited interventions than others (e.g., psychoanalysis, person-centred counselling, and Gestalt therapy).

Techniques used to achieve the goals are also important. For example, if the counsellor is employing a behavioural or developmental approach, it is often necessary to be in a position to structure the client's environment to achieve the counselling objectives. Similarly, counsellors who are using a trait-and-factor approach must not only have a variety of psychometric and other data available about the client, they must also be skilled in interpreting, integrating, and implementing assessment results. One cannot implement any approach successfully unless the necessary resources are available.

An additional consideration is whether the approach is amenable to measurement of change in the client's behaviour. Counsellors live in an age of accountability and must, therefore, be able to demonstrate their effectiveness. Whereas some approaches (e.g., behavioural and trait-and-factor) offer rather concrete and easily measured criteria for success (e.g., number of hours spent studying, number of widgets produced, whether the client is successfully placed or not), other approaches such as psychoanalytic, person-centred, and the developmental approaches to career choice offer much more complex and difficult to measure criteria (e.g., strength of the ego, self-actualization, and career maturity). Thus, the extent to which counsellors must demonstrate their effectiveness to an external funding body may significantly affect the approach which the counsellors decide to use.

A useful summary of these considerations is provided by Thomas, Butler, and Parker (1987):

> A final and global consideration is the relevance
> and appropriateness of a counselling approach for
> rehabilitation. This judgment stems from both the

sum and the crossproducts of the factors cited. The approach selected should ideally be congruent with the basic philosophy and theoretical orientation of the counsellor; be congruent with his or her training and personality; be applicable to the clients of the agency; be directed to goals acceptable to the client, counsellor, and the agency; and in general mesh well with the specific rehabilitation context. No single approach has yet been blessed with a consensus of endorsements. The onus is upon the student and practitioner to apply their training, experience, and professional judgment to select an approach that best suits their unique responsibilities. (p.72).

This chapter presents an overview of the major theories of counselling and psychotherapy and career development and occupational choice. The specific approaches to counselling and psychotherapy discussed are as follows: Psychodynamic, including drive/structure and relational structure approaches; Humanistic, including person-centred therapy and Gestalt therapy; Cognitive, including trait-and-factor counselling, rational-emotive therapy, and reality therapy; and Behavioural, including behavioural counselling, Dollard and Miller's reinforcement theory, and Wolpe's psychotherapy by reciprocal inhibition. Three categories of career development and occupational choice theories are also discussed: Personality based theories, including Roe's personality theory of occupational choice and Holland's career typology theory; Developmental theories, including Super's developmental self-concept theory, Ginzberg, Ginsburg, Axelrad and Herma's developmental theory of occupational choice, and Tiedeman's developmental career decision making theory; and two rehabilitation theories, which are the Minnesota Theory of Work Adjustment and McMahon's Model of Vocational Redevelopment. In each case, the emphasis of the discussion is on how rehabilitation practitioners can use the theory to improve their practice.

THEORIES OF COUNSELLING AND PSYCHOTHERAPY

Psychodynamic Approaches

Psychodynamic approaches to counselling and psychotherapy had their origins in the early works of Jerome Breuer and Sigmund Freud (1893-95). From a rehabilitation perspective, it is interesting that virtually all of the patients described by Breuer and Freud in their classic *Studies on Hysteria* monograph displayed marked physical symptoms (e.g., Anna O., Fraulein Elisabeth von R.). While Breuer abandoned psychoanalysis (and Freud) in 1894 due to his discomfort with the "transference" relationship which eventually developed between him and Anna O., and his reluctance to be identified with Freud's ideas about the sexual origins of psychopathology, Freud continued to develop the theories and techniques of psychoanalysis until his death in 1939.

Initially, Breuer and Freud used the technique of hypnosis to help patients remember and abreact early conflictual situations to relieve their hysterical symptoms. Later, because he found the effects of hypnosis limited and did not consider himself to be a good hypnotist, Freud would place his hand on the patient's head and order her to remember. Eventually, he relied on the technique of free association, which became the fundamental rule of psychoanalysis. Although Freud published mountains of theoretical papers, case studies, letters, etc., on psychoanalysis, he wrote only six papers on the technique, which at the time he believed should be only for the eyes of analysts.

Freud's theories of psychoanalysis went through several revisions, but he also retained some key elements along the way. Among the more important concepts were the existence of drives (instincts), the topographical theory (i.e., the existence of the systems conscious, preconscious, and unconscious), the dual-instinct theory [sex (libido, Eros) and aggression (death instinct, Thanatos)], and the structure theory (id, ego, and superego). Two other important concepts were the psychosexual stages (oral, anal, phallic, latent, and genital) and the critical idea of the Oedipal complex and associated concepts such as castration anxiety and penis envy.

Techniques used by Freud and by modern analysts of

more orthodox persuasion include: free association, the neutral stance, dream analysis, the interpretation of resistance, and the working through of the "transference neurosis". While at least some of Freud's theories and related concepts are accepted by a majority of classical analysts, many other analysts, both during Freud's time and to the present, reject many of Freud's ideas.

Controversies, even among analysts, concern essentially the primacy of the drives as well as the importance of Oedipal (ages 3-6) vs. pre-Oedipal origins of pathology. For Freud, psychopathology was related to intrapsychic conflict arising from sexual and aggressive issues during the Oedipal period. Modern theorists such as Heinz Kohut, Otto Kernberg, Margaret Mahler, and D.W. Winnicott place more emphasis on early object relations and developmental problems. Essentially, the question is whether emotional disturbance is the result of conflicts between the individual's instincts and society-at-large or whether pathology results primarily from developmental deficits.

Obviously, how one views the development of pathology will influence the types of interventions selected. Classical theorists emphasize the "neutral" stance, interpretation of transference and resistance, dream analysis, and free association; whereas object relation theorists place more emphasis on the real relationship, countertransference interpretations, empathy, and the creation of what Winnicott calls a "holding environment". In many respects, modern psychoanalytic theorists are similar to person-centred therapists in their emphasis on the development of the self, empathy, the real relationship, and the creation of a facilitative therapeutic environment. However, there are vast differences between the two groups in how they view the origin and nature of psychopathology as well as how they view the treatment environment. In the case of both drive/structure and relational/structure theorists, a major goal of therapy with persons with disabilities would logically be to strengthen the ego and improve self-esteem (Cubbage and Thomas, 1989).

Several concepts from psychoanalytic theory can be used in the everyday practice of rehabilitation counsellors. According to Cook (1987), psychoanalytic conceptualizations of the ego defences (e.g., A. Freud, 1936; Freud, 1923) are especially useful to understanding the impact of disability on the individual. Cook

41

listed four defense mechanisms which are continually referred to in the literature on adjustment to physical disability: repression, projection, reaction formation, and regression. Cubbage and Thomas (1989) expanded this list to include denial, compensation, displacement, sublimation, restriction of the ego, and rationalization. A discussion of these issues is also provided by Krueger (1984). By recognizing the role that defense mechanisms play in adjustment to disability, the rehabilitation counsellor is in a better position not only to understand the client's behaviour, but also to capitalize on those defenses which are being positively used to promote coping.

Other classical psychoanalytic concepts which may have particular relevance to work with persons with a disability are castration anxiety, fear of loss of love, narcissism, the concept of secondary gain, and the death instinct. For a more detailed discussion of these issues, see Cubbage and Thomas (1989). The reader is also referred to Siller (1988) for a discussion of intrapsychic aspects of attitudes toward persons with a disability.

As a final observation, it should be noted that modern psychoanalytic theorists emphasize the importance of the integrity of the self and the specific role of empathy in the healing process (Kohut, 1984). Also presented are observations on the importance of creating what is called a "holding environment" to enable patients to mend what have essentially been narcissistic injuries of the past (Winnicott, 1975). By offering empathy and creating what might loosely be called the holding environment advocated by Winnicott, rehabilitation counsellors could be important instruments in facilitating what would probably be, without impingement from the environment, a natural healing process (Thomas and McGinnis, in press).

Humanistic Approaches

Humanistic approaches are based on a common fundamental belief in the client as the active agent of change in the context of an interpersonal relationship that stresses the uniqueness of the individual's own experience. Client feelings and emotions, rather than behaviour or beliefs are stressed. The counsellor's role is to facilitate a warm and empathic environment in which clients are given the freedom to explore themselves; given such an environment, clients can successfully redirect their own lives. Two approaches, person-centred therapy and Gestalt therapy, will be reviewed under this classification.

Person-centred therapy, initially called client-centred counselling, originated with Carl Rogers (1942, 1951, 1961). It has been extended through the writings and research of a number of associates and followers, as documented by Bergin and Garfield (1971), Carkhuff and Berenson (1977), and Kiesler (1973). Person-centred counselling developed out of a reaction against psychoanalytic therapy, resulting in philosophical and theoretical foundations that differ significantly from those espoused by Freud.

Human beings are viewed as innately good, realistic, and forward moving. In his well-developed theory of personality and development, Rogers recognized several innate components that include:

1. The actualizing tendency, which is an inherent proclivity of the individual to develop capabilities in ways that serve to enhance the individual;
2. The tendency toward self-actualization, which is a general tendency of the individual toward actualization in that component of experience of the individual that is symbolized in the self;
3. Awareness and symbolization, representing the capacity to perceive situational events and internal stimuli, and to represent the awareness in symbolic form; and
4. The organizing principle that integrates new experiences with past behaviour and experience.

A fully functioning individual symbolizes his or her experiences accurately in awareness. Since needs for positive regard from others and positive self-regard are readily fulfilled, the fully functioning person is free of threat and defensiveness. Experience is not distorted or denied to awareness. In contrast, under conditions of less than optimal functioning, the individual senses a lack of congruence between self and experience; is defensive, anxious, and lacks positive self-regard; and tends to deny, ignore, or distort the perception of discrepant responses.

The goal of counselling of this approach is for clients to become self-actualized through the development of all capacities that serve to maintain or enhance the self. Specific goals of counselling are determined by the clients, who are assumed capable of moving toward positive mental health. Potential positive outcomes from the process of therapy include greater congruence, openness of experience, reduction of defensiveness, and more realistic, objective, and comprehensive perceptions. As a further result of successful person-centred counselling, clients become more effective in problem solving, acquire a more positive self-regard, and sense the real self as more congruent with the ideal self. Finally, clients perceive their own behaviour as being under their self-control (Meador and Rogers, 1984).

Counselling techniques primarily involve reflection of client feelings and the creation of the facilitative conditions of the therapeutic process. The necessary and sufficient conditions of therapeutic change identified by Rogers may be summarized as follows:

1. Two persons are in contact;
2. One, the client, is in a state of incongruence, being vulnerable or anxious;
3. The other person, the therapist, is congruent in the relationship;
4. The therapist experiences unconditional positive regard toward the client;
5. The therapist experiences an accurate empathic understanding of the client's internal frame of reference;
6. The client perceives, at least to a minimum degree, conditions 4 and 5 (Patterson, 1986, p. 389).

The process of therapy, then, is described not in terms of specific rules, but as a logical outcome of the conditions just listed and the basic assumptions concerning personality change. During the process, the client becomes more open to experiencing feelings, more aware of incongruence between experience and self, and more aware of feelings that were previously denied to awareness or distorted.

The counsellor is expected to experience and communicate congruence (genuineness), unconditional positive regard (acceptance), and accurate empathy (understanding). Giving advice or suggestions of alternative solutions, interpretation, probing, role-playing or information-giving, admonishment, or other intrusions of the counsellor's values are regarded as detrimental to client growth. Counsellor introduction of psychometric test data, occupational information, or case history material is similarly renounced.

Criteria for change are implied by the expected outcomes of this therapy. In operationalizing the expected outcomes for purposes of research, client self-report techniques are most consistent with the underlying philosophy of person-centred counselling. The most commonly used techniques of assessment in research are measures of self-concept and indices of congruence between real and ideal self. Application of person-centred therapy to rehabilitation settings has been controversial. Serious questions have been raised about its appropriateness for clients with limited intelligence and/or limited verbal ability, particularly those who are labelled mentally retarded or severely psychotic. Rogers, however, reversed his original dictum against using his approaches with people who are retarded. In addition, he also conducted extensive research on the effectiveness of person-centred counselling with individuals diagnosed as schizophrenic (Rogers, Gendlin, Kiesler, and Truax, 1967).

Because this approach emphasizes the importance of personal attributes (which may or may not be modified by education) rather than formal training in psychotherapy, adoption of the approach is possible for many rehabilitation counsellors. The goals of therapy may conflict with those set by some service agencies. Perhaps most important in this regard is the potential role conflict for counsellors, particularly those in governmental agencies who are required to set goals, assess vocational competencies, provide occupational information, and make decisions concerning eligibility for, and provision of, rehabilitation services. Another criticism is that extensive counselling time is required.

Gestalt therapy is generally attributed to Fritz Perls, with the books by Perls (1969) and Perls, Hefferline, and Goodman (1951) being regarded as landmark publications. The approach, which is based upon Gestalt psychology, emphasizes approaching individuals from a holistic rather than an analytic framework. In developing Gestalt therapy, Perls also drew upon psychoanalysis and existential philosophy. A major concept from Gestalt psychology is the perceptual field that represents the context and extent of an individual's perceptions. The individual is viewed as striving to organize stimuli into wholes. This organization is accomplished in the context of figure-ground relationships, the figure constituting the immediate needs and the activities associated with meeting these needs and the ground with the physical and psychological surrounds. As shifts in stimuli occur, a Gestalt or unified understanding is formed. Somewhat simplistically, people's abilities to shift, meet needs, and form complete Gestalts are related to their complete and accurate awareness of both figure and ground. Anything that detracts from comprehensive and accurate awareness interferes with people's capacities to act effectively as fully functioning people.

According to Passons (1975, p. 14), Gestalt therapy is based on the following assumptions:

1. [A human being] is a whole who is (rather than has) a body, emotions, thoughts, sensations, and perceptions, all of which function interrelatedly;
2. [A human being] is a part of his (or her) environment and cannot be understood outside of it;
3. [Human beings are] proactive rather than reactive. [They] determine [their] own responses to external and proprioceptive stimuli;
4. [Human beings are] capable of being aware of [their] sensations, thoughts, emotions, and perceptions;
5. [A human being], through self-awareness, is capable of choice and is thus responsible for covert and overt behaviour;
6. [Human beings possess] the wherewithal and resources to live effectively and to restore [themselves] through [their] own assets;
7. [Human beings] can experience [themselves] only in the present. The past and the future can be experienced only in the now through remembering and anticipation;
8. [A human being] is neither intrinsically good nor bad;

An important concept in understanding personality development is what Perls referred to as the ego boundary. At an early age children learn to differentiate what is within themselves and what is outside. During development the self and self-image are formed, the self being what the individual really is and the self-image reflecting the expectations of others.

Growth is characterized by contact, sensing, excitement, and formation of gestalts. Frustration facilitates growth in that it encourages people to mobilize resources and act on their own. Fully functioning people are those who are comprehensively aware of their senses, can fully express themselves, have no major "incomplete" life experiences, are self-supporting, and are not maintaining self-images incongruent with the self (Simkin and Yontif, 1984).

The goal of Gestalt therapy is the integration of the individual with all the portions of experience that have been disowned to the point that the client is self-directive. The major intermediate goal is increased awareness because only with increased awareness can the "unfinished business" of life be recognized and confronted.

Perls (1969), Kempler (1973) and Polster and Polster (1973) have proposed a wide range of techniques, all of which emphasize experiencing an awareness in the "here and now." Counsellors are active, confrontative, probing, and authoritative. The role-playing, the "hot seat," dream review, and client fantasizing techniques, which are a number of the commonly acceptable approaches in Gestalt therapy, are designed to facilitate clients to fully experience concerns, feelings, attitudes, or disowned aspects of themselves. Nonverbal behaviour is considered significant: the bowed head or clenched fist is challenged to encourage clients to share the associated feelings. Frustration is used to discourage dependency, mobilize resources, and encourage expression of feeling. Intensive group workshops are often used for the emotional impact and elicitation of awareness. See Levitsky and Perls (1970) for a comprehensive listing of "rules" and "games" of Gestalt therapy.

Methods for assessing constructs of client change are elusive and subjective in Gestalt therapy. One such construct, level of goal attainment, is assessed primarily through clinical judgment largely because appropriate objective measures of change have not been developed. Consequently, this and other approaches to evaluating the outcomes of Gestalt therapy have not been verified by research.

Implications for rehabilitation do not differ significantly from those cited for person-centred therapy. Gestalt therapy has been used with children, adolescents, adults, alcoholics, emotionally disturbed people, and mentally retarded people. Commonly treated problems include generalized anxiety, discomfort, psychosomatic disorders, and *anomie*. It is an appropriate therapy modality for clients who have difficulty in interpersonal relationships, as well as those with distorted or limiting self-images. Counsellor requirements are not as precisely specified as in the person-centred approach, but clearly the counsellor should be capable of a dynamic and active role in the counselling relationship. In view of the typical level of risk-taking with clients, extensive training and personal therapy are required for recognition as a Gestalt therapist.

Cognitive Approaches

In contrast to humanistic approaches, which focus on client feelings, experiencing, and awareness, cognitive approaches emphasize a logical and intellectual solution of the client's problems. The two approaches presented here, trait-factor counselling and rational-emotive therapy, have different historical precedents and generally have focussed on different clientele. They are grouped together somewhat arbitrarily based on their "cognitive" emphasis. Reality therapy is also briefly discussed under this same rubric.

The major spokesman for *trait-factor counselling* was Edmund G. Williamson (1950, 1965), although it represented a point of view shared by a number of his colleagues at the University of Minnesota. Unlike Rogers and Perls, whose views stemmed from a reaction against the clinical application of psychoanalysis, Williamson's viewpoint appeared to have developed from his lifelong interest in vocational guidance and counselling. Unlike all others cited in the counselling and psychotherapy section of this book, it is the only approach that emerged from vocational counselling and emphasizes educational and vocational adjustment. In addition, it stresses the use of psychological testing in the counselling process.

A basic assumption of the trait-factor approach is that each individual is born with the potential for both good and evil.

Individuals strive to develop their full potential, which may be viewed as excellence in all aspects of human development. But, quite important to this approach, the individual needs assistance from others to realize the fullest of this potential. Development is more likely to be fostered by rational processes than by an affective or intuitive capacity. Assumptions more directly related to counselling itself include the following:

1. Major traits of the individual are measurable and can be used to match an individual to a vocation or job;
2. Information derived from the individual in testing and diagnostic interviewing can be used in decision-making concerning vocational and general life adjustment;
3. Information derived from the individual must be considered in the light of demands made in the environment;
4. A major task in counselling is the systematic synthesis of information so that reasonable predictions can be made about the individual's "fit" with the job and other important dimensions of the environment;

The goal of counselling is broad: to assist clients toward optimal development in all aspects of their personalities. Considerable stress is placed on social enlightenment, self-understanding, and self-direction rather than on autonomous individuation. The client is expected to be a responsible member of society and conform to its mores and values.

Techniques of counselling are not fully explicated, but the steps in the counselling process have been rather clearly delineated as follows:

1. Analysis, the initial step, involves the systematic collection of data and information about the client to acquire an understanding of the client's problem and the demands of current and future adjustment. Specific tools will vary with the setting, but they include the initial interview, case history, medical history, and psychological tests. From these are derived family history, health history, educational and work history, and an overview of social, avocational and vocational interests and objectives;
2. Synthesis is the summarizing and organizing of data to

determine the client's assets, liabilities, adjustments, and maladjustments;

3. Diagnosis pertains to the summary of problems and their causes. Unlike medical diagnosis, which is almost solely the practitioner's responsibility, diagnosis involves the client's participation to the extent of his or her intellectual and emotional capabilities;

4. Prognosis refers to the counsellor's specific predictions of probable outcomes, given a variety of possible courses of action and other contingencies;

5. Counselling is viewed as that phase in which the counsellor assists the client in utilizing internal and external resources to achieve optimum adjustment. It involves a process of guided re-education. Five categories of techniques have been identified, including forcing conformity, changing the environment, selecting the appropriate environment, learning needed skills, and changing attitudes. These are general headings; specific techniques vary with the individual client and the presenting problem. Some common threads throughout include establishing rapport, cultivating self-understanding, and advising or planning a programme of action. The counsellor is active in the process, avoids being dogmatic, but may offer advice and information freely, while encouraging the client to express and bring out ideas. Direct assistance in implementing the plan is proffered when necessary, and the counsellor will involve others as deemed appropriate;

6. Follow-up is not fully explicated, but implies availability of the counsellor to deal with recurring problems and to determine whether the counselling has been effective.

Since the approach has been used extensively in the university setting, educational and vocational successes have been cited as appropriate measures of change. Client satisfaction and "satisfactoriness" on the job, measurement constructs developed in the Minnesota Studies on Vocational Rehabilitation (Dawis, 1967), could be logically used in this approach as indices of effectiveness.

A major counsellor requirement is the ability to interpret psychological test results and to understand the merits and liabilities of psychological measurement. Goals of counselling are generally congruent with the broader goals of rehabilitation. Techniques are usually well within the repertoire of skills of most rehabilitation counsellors and deemed appropriate in most settings. Some counsellors, however, will have difficulty in accepting the philosophical underpinnings of this approach. Moreover, the emphasis on the use of psychometric tests and other assessment techniques could be a significant disadvantage of the trait-factor approach given the spurious validity characteristics of many of these techniques when applied to people with disabilities.

Rational-emotive therapy (RET) was developed by Albert Ellis who, like Rogers and Perls, reacted negatively to psychoanalysis. His approach emerged from his clinical practice which was primarily in sex and marital counselling.

A key to understanding RET is the so-called A-B-C paradigm: "When a highly charged emotional consequence (C) follows a significant activating event (A), A may be seen to, but does not actually cause C. Instead, emotional consequences are largely created by B, the individual's belief system" (Ellis, 1984, p. 196). In other words, it is not what happens that causes difficulty and stress, but the person's irrational beliefs about what has happened. If these beliefs can be rationally challenged and disputed, the undesirable emotional consequences will cease.

A succinct statement of the goals of therapy must be inferred; essentially, it is to eliminate emotional disturbance by substituting rational beliefs and thinking for the irrationality. As a result of successful RET, clients become more independent of the evaluations of others and rely more on positive self-reinforcement for their behaviour.

Conventional techniques used in psychoanalytic and humanistic approaches to therapy are avoided. The client is discouraged from relating past history, abreacting, or free associating. Ellis views free association, dream analysis, dynamically oriented interpretation, reassurance, and the like as inefficient and irrelevant. Generally, the therapist uses an active and directive approach to identify the core of irrational ideas that underlie the disturbed behaviour, challenges the client to logically defend those ideas, and directively shows that they do not work. Rational substitutes are introduced, and the client is taught how to sequence the substitutes. Homework assignments are often made in which the client may listen to cassette recordings of the previous session or record situations between sessions in which irrational beliefs have been assailed.

Criteria for success of the approach are couched in general terms, and include reduced anxiousness and defensiveness, increased skills in attacking irrational beliefs and enhancing reality testing, greater levels of individuality and freedom of choice, and heightened self-confidence and self-acceptance (Ellis, 1984). These criteria have been operationally defined primarily by therapist report. However, researchers have developed rational behaviour scales that show promise for assessing the effectiveness of the approach (e.g., see Shorkey and Whiteman, 1977).

Applicability of RET to rehabilitation settings may be evaluated from a number of viewpoints. It does not appear to be feasible for individuals with low intelligence levels or thought disorders associated with brain damage. It does not appear to be effective in educational and vocational decision-making, but is more appropriate when low self-esteem, poor social skills, or lack of acceptance of disability interfere with this process, or when the client is overwhelmed by the transition from the hospital or institution to the community. And finally, the didactic and directive aspects of RET would blend reasonably well with most rehabilitation counsellor training programmes.

One other cognitive approach, *Reality therapy*, should be briefly noted. Reality therapy, a relative newcomer to the field of psychological treatment, was introduced by Glasser (1965, 1969). Glasser (1984, p. 320) describes Reality therapy as being

> applicable to individuals with any sort of psychological problem ... It focusses on the present and upon getting people to understand that they choose essentially all their actions in an attempt to fulfill basic needs...The therapists's task is to lead them toward... more responsible choices.

In the counselling process, the counsellor is verbally active, sets limits, is guided by a precise behaviour contract with the client, and may engage in a wide variety of interactional techniques (e.g., confrontation and constructive arguing) to direct the client toward the realities of the present and the immediate future. The focus is on behaviours, not feelings, and particularly on how clients will act in a responsible manner on their own behalf.

The therapist's goal is to increase responsible client behaviour. According to Glasser, a responsible behaviour is one that satisfies one's needs without preventing others from satisfying theirs. The therapist may become didactic when clients need assistance in making effective choices, and does not accept excuses or condone punishment.

Reality therapy has not yet been widely used in rehabilitation settings, but it does appear to have potential value for those with "responsibility" problems - for example, the public offender, the drug or alcohol abuser, and the overly dependent client. Although the basic tenets have been thoroughly documented, little research has been conducted to verify their utility.

Behavioural Approaches

Behavioural approaches may be extended to include counselling strategies which involve learning-theory principles and focus on change of behaviour rather than feelings, attitudes, or beliefs, but do involve a therapist-client relationship rather than an impersonal behaviour management paradigm. One approach has been selected for more detailed review, Krumboltz' behavioural counselling. Two others, Dollard and Miller's marriage of reinforcement and psychoanalytic theories, and Wolpe's psychotherapy by reciprocal inhibition will also be briefly noted.

Behavioural counselling was developed initially for counselling services in the public school setting by John Krumboltz and a number of associates at Stanford University. Basic references include Krumboltz and Thoreson (1969; 1976) and Hosford and de Visser (1974). Highly eclectic in the use of techniques, its theoretical principles stem primarily from learning theory. Basic concepts include the following:

1. People have equal potentialities for good and evil;
2. People are capable of change;
3. Each person has unique problems that must be appreciated on an individual basis;

4. Behaviour is guided by external conditions that are interpreted by the individual's cognitive processes.

There is little preoccupation with the causality and classification of maladaptive behaviour, and no assumptions are made about psychopathological processes. Current problems may stem from either learned maladaptive behaviour or failure to have learned specific adaptive behaviours. Consequently, the focus is on identifying the client's current problem, establishing specific behavioural goals to alleviate the problem, and selecting the most appropriate techniques to achieve the goal.

Krumboltz and Thoresen (1969) identified four general types of client problems:

1. Deficient decision-making skills;
2. Ineffective academic (vocationally-related) skills;
3. Inappropriate social skills;
4. Self-defeating fears and anxieties.

Essential features include four interrelated characteristics that enable behavioural counsellors to respond flexibly and adapt new, continuously improving procedures to help their clients. The first concerns the process of formulating counselling goals. Of all the major approaches, behavioural counselling places the greatest emphasis on the process of goal formulation. A goal should meet three essential criteria:

1. It must be desired by the client;
2. The counsellor must be willing to help the client achieve the goal;
3. It must be possible to assess the extent to which the client achieves the goal (Krumboltz, 1966).

A second feature is that the same technique is not universally applied. A procedure or combination of procedures is elected to help clients accomplish their unique goals. Third, there are no restrictions on the possible techniques to be used, except those imposed by ethical considerations. There is no recommended approved list; counsellors are encouraged to experiment and systematically explore new techniques, provided, of course, these are within their repertoire of skills.

Finally, procedures need to be modified and changed on the basis of empirical evidence.

Three classifications of goals are recognized: altering or diminishing maladaptive behaviour, learning the decision-making process, and preventing problems. The latter includes the acquisition of new behaviours (e.g., job-seeking skills) that will be needed to prevent difficulties in the future.

Because of the wide range of continually evolving techniques used with this approach, no single listing is feasible (see Krumboltz and Thoresen [1969, 1976] for a comprehensive overview that includes reinforcement techniques such as simulation and planning). Certain traditional procedures that focus primarily on feelings, experiencing, and insight, while not expressly "forbidden", do not logically fit the system. One procedural element common to most techniques is the written behavioural contract in which the commitments of the client and counsellor toward achievement of the goal are clearly identified.

Criteria for success under this approach tend to be unique to each client. Generally, these can be defined as the acquisition of adaptive behaviour or extinction of problem behaviour as reported by the counsellor, the client, or significant others.

The approach appears to be applicable to a wide range of rehabilitation settings and clientele. No categories of clients are arbitrarily excluded. Presenting problems of substantial numbers of rehabilitation clients (e.g., absence of job-seeking and maintaining skills, inappropriate social behaviours, and fears related to changing vocations) appear to be amenable to behavioural counselling. Counsellors would require special training in the application of techniques based on the learning theory model as well as training in the skills of problem identification and goal formulation. Techniques that require cooperation of others, such as maintaining reinforcement contingencies, may set some limits on application.

Among the other behaviour therapy approaches, two warrant brief mention. The approach of Dollard and Miller (1950) is of particular interest because of their attempt to integrate learning theory and psychoanalysis, but their explanation of behaviour change is couched primarily in learning theory terminology. For a recent summary of their approach, see Patterson (1986).

Joseph Wolpe (1958, 1969) developed his psychotherapy by reciprocal inhibition approach mainly from studies of experimental neuroses in animals. In his investigations, he induced neurotic reactions in cats and found the reactions could be reduced by conditioned inhibition. The basic concept, reciprocal inhibition, refers to the elimination or weakening of responses, such as anxiety or fear, through the process of conditioning. Specific techniques include systematic desensitization, assertiveness training, aversion therapy, therapeutic sexual arousal, and operant conditioning methods.

CAREER DEVELOPMENT AND OCCUPATIONAL CHOICE THEORIES

Personality-Based Theories

Two widely respected theories, developed by Anne Roe and John Holland, suggest that occupational behaviour is influenced primarily by personality variables. Roe (1956) based her theory on Maslow's (1954) need hierarchy and on speculations regarding the process through which genetic predispositions and parent-child relationships affect later career development. Furthermore, she constructed an occupational classification system consisting of the following eight groups and six levels:

GROUPS		LEVELS	
I.	Service	1.	Professional and Managerial
II.	Business Contact	2.	Professional and Managerial
III.	Managerial	3.	Semiprofessional
IV.	Technology	4.	Skilled
V.	Outdoor	5.	Semiskilled
VI.	Science	6.	Unskilled
VII.	General Cultural		
VIII.	Arts and Entertainment		

(National Occupational Information Coordinating Committee, 1986)

Roe believed that an individual's career development increasingly focussed on one of the six levels due to the individual's ability level and socioeconomic background, and on one of the eight occupational groups due to the influence of early childhood experiences. Roe postulated that the emotional climate of the home, which is characterized by the relationship between parent and child, shapes the individual's personality. The home's emotional climate can be concurrently described as either warm or cold and as belonging to one of three major types of parent-child relationships (each with two subtypes): acceptance of the child (loving or casual), avoidance of the child (neglecting or rejecting), or emotional concentration on the child (overprotective or overdemanding). The home's emotional climate determines the child's orientation toward persons. Specifically, individual's from *loving, overprotecting,* or *overdemanding* homes tend to have a *major orientation toward persons.* Those experiencing *casual acceptance, neglect,* or *rejection* tend to possess a *major orientation away from persons.* And finally, individuals select occupations based on their orientation toward or away from persons. Person-oriented occupational areas include Service, Business Contact, Managerial, General Culture, and Arts and Entertainment; nonperson-oriented areas include Technology, Outdoors, and Science (Isaacson, 1985).

Researchers testing Roe's theory generally have failed to find supportive evidence (Isaacson, 1985; Osipow, 1983; Zunker, 1986). Clearly, the pivotal aspects of her theory are difficult to measure accurately. The emotional climate of the home has been determined through retrospective self-report, and thus may suffer limited reliability and validity. Additional problems have resulted from difficulty in controlling for the many nuisance and contaminating variables. Finally, thorough testing of Roe's hypotheses, which would require painstaking longitudinal data collection, has not been pursued because of the time and expense involved (Isaacson, 1985; Zunker, 1986).

In contrast to Roe, Holland did not focus upon early experiences or parent-child relationships in formulating his theory of occupational choice. Instead, he placed emphasis on the influence of a person's personality type in determining vocational choice. The principle underlying Holland's theory is that vocational choice is an expression of personality (Holland, 1985a). Four assumptions undergird his theory:

1. Most people in our culture have one of six modal personal styles or personality types — realistic (R), investigative (I), artistic (A), social (S), enterprising (E) or conventional (C);
2. Vocational environments likewise can be classified into the same six types — realistic, investigative, artistic, social, enterprising, or conventional;
3. People search for vocational environments that allow them to express their abilities, attitudes, values, and preferred roles;
4. An individual's vocational behaviour is determined by the interaction between his or her personality and the characteristics of the work environment (Holland, 1966, 1973).

   A person's personality type can be measured through using a number of instruments, for example, the *Self Directed Search* and *Vocational Preference Inventory*. Using these instruments allows one to assign a three-letter code (e.g., RIC) to indicate an individual's personality type. Jobs can also be coded according to the three-letter scheme using the Dictionary of Holland Occupational Codes (Gottfriedson, Holland, and Ogawa, 1982). Finally, one can attempt to match the personality code to job codes to determine the goodness of fit between personality and work environment.

   In addition to the above four assumptions, Holland (1985b) posed three supplementary propositions:
5. The degree of congruence between an individual's personality and his or her vocational environment can be gauged by an hexagonal model (see Figure 3.1). The shorter the distance between a person's personality type and his or her occupational environment type, the greater the congruence or fit. For instance, an individual with a realistic personality and a realistic environment would lie on the same point on the hexagon, indicating the greatest degree of congruence. A person with a realistic personality and a social environment would be most incongruent because the R and S points on the hexagon are furthest apart.

Figure 3.1: Holland's hexagonal model showing the distance between the realistic and other five personality types.

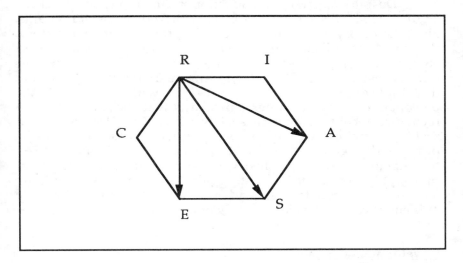

6. The degree of consistency *within* a person or a vocational environment can also be estimated using the hexagonal model. Adjacent types on the model are most consistent (e.g., R and I, R and C, E and C, E and S, etc.), while opposite types are least consistent (e.g., R and S, C and A, and E and I). A person who had a two-letter code of RS or CA or EI would indicate an inconsistency because the codes reflect opposing orientations, attitudes, and preferences.

7. The degree of differentiation of an individual or environment may vary significantly. For example, a person or an environment may most closely resemble one of the six types, or may resemble several types. The former person or environment would be termed differentiated, while the latter would be labelled undifferentiated. Furthermore, highly differentiated people would likely be described well by Holland's theoretical model. Additionally, Holland (1973) suggests a positive relationship between degree of

differentiation and a person's age and level of crystallization of vocational goals.

Despite receiving broad support in numerous research studies, Holland's theory has been criticized on several counts. First, the theory is primarily descriptive, rather than explanatory. Emphasis is placed on describing both personality and environment types, perhaps at the expense of explaining the critical causal factors determining personality types and developmental sequences through which individuals' personalities pass. Another criticism is that the theory fails to recognize recent changes in society which have led to women seeking a wider variety of occupational roles, and thus is purportedly gender biased (Isaacson, 1985; Zunker, 1986). Nonetheless, Holland's theory is without question the most thoroughly researched, most highly developed in providing measures of constructs, and probably the most broadly influential career development theory today.

Developmental Theories

One of the most productive lines of inquiry into how individuals make vocational choices is the developmental approach. This approach, which is exemplified especially by Super's developmental self-concept theory, had its origins in the early 1950's (Ginzberg, Ginsburg, Axelrad, and Herma 1951; Super, 1953). Probably the most distinguishing characteristic of this approach is the idea that when developing vocationally and in making occupational choices, individuals pass through various developmental stages and that specific developmental tasks are associated with these various stages. The three most prominent of the developmental theories are presented by Donald Super (1953; 1957; 1964; 1969; 1980; 1984), Eli Ginzberg and his associates (Ginzberg, 1952; 1970; 1972; 1984; Ginzberg et al., 1951) and David Tiedeman and his associates (O'Hara and Tiedeman, 1959; Tiedeman, 1961; 1979; Tiedeman and O'Hara, 1963; Tiedeman and Miller-Tiedeman, 1979, 1984).

Of the three approaches listed above, Super's is clearly the most visible and has accumulated the largest amount of research support. The theory is presented in the form of 12 propositions

(Super, 1984). These propositions are as follows:

1. People differ in their abilities, interests, and personalities;
2. People are qualified, by virtue of these characteristics, each for a number of occupations;
3. Each of these occupations requires a characteristic pattern of abilities, interests, and personality traits, with tolerances wide enough to allow both some variety of occupations for each individual and some variety of individuals in each occupation;
4. Vocational preferences and competencies, the situations in which people live and work, and hence their self-concepts, change with time and experience, although self-concepts are generally fairly stable from late adolescence until late maturity, making choice and adjustment a continuous process;
5. This process of change may be summed up in a series of life stages (or "maxicycles") characterized as those of growth, exploration, establishment, maintenance, and decline, and these stages may in turn be subdivided into (a) the fantasy, tentative, and realistic phases of the exploratory stage and (b) the trial and stable phases of the establishment stage. A smaller cycle takes place in transitions from one stage to the next or each time an unstable or multiple-trial career is unstabilized, which involves new growth, re-exploration, and re-establishment;
6. The nature of the career pattern - that is, the occupational level attained and the sequence, frequency, and duration of trial and stable jobs – is determined by the individual's parental socioeconomic level, mental ability, and personality characteristics, and by the opportunities to which he or she is exposed;
7. Development through the life stages can be guided, partly by facilitating the maturing of abilities and interests and partly by aiding in reality testing and in the development of self-concepts;
8. The process of career development is essentially that of developing and implementing self-concepts; it is a synthesizing and compromising process in which the self-concept is a product of the interaction of inherited

aptitudes, physical make-up, opportunity to play various roles, and evaluations of the extent to which the results of role playing meet with the approval of superiors and fellows;

9. The process of synthesis or of compromise between individual and social factors, between self-concept and reality, is one of role playing, whether the role is played in fantasy, in the counselling interview, or in real-life activities such as classes, clubs, part-time work, and entry jobs;

10. Work satisfactions and life satisfactions depend on the extent to which the individual finds adequate outlets for abilities, interests, personality traits, and values; they depend on establishment in a type of work, a work situation, and a way of life in which one can play the kind of role that growth and exploratory experiences have led one to consider congenial and appropriate (Super, 1953, pp. 189-190);

11. The degree of satisfaction people attain from work is proportionate to the degree to which they have been able to implement self-concepts;

12. Work and occupation provide a focus for personality organization for most men and many women, although for some persons this focus is peripheral, incidental, or even nonexistent, and other foci, such as leisure activities and homemaking, are central (Super and Bachrach, 1957, pp. 11-12). (Social traditions, such as sex-role stereotyping, racial and ethnic biases, and the opportunity structure as well as individual differences are important determinants of preferences for roles such as those of worker, leisurite and homemaker; pp. 194-196.)

Three major streams of thought influenced Super in the derivation of his theory (Osipow, 1983): (a) differential psychology; (b) developmental psychology (especially the work of Charlotte Buehler (1933) on life stages); and (c) the self-concept and personal construct theories of Rogers (1951) and Snygg and Combs (1949). While at least one prominent rehabilitation theorist (Neff, 1985) has severely criticized Super for the emphasis placed in his theory on the development of the self-concept, it is this aspect of the theory which has received the most research support and which, in conjunction with his developmental perspective, has gained the most support from counsellors. Essentially, Super believes that occupational choice represents the implementation of the individual's self-concepts and that the development of these self-concepts is a process which is governed and influenced by the passage through various life stages. By intervening at these various stages, counsellors can positively influence and assist clients to clarify their vocational self-concepts by providing for exploratory activities and helping to clarify interests, values, and abilities.

From a rehabilitation counselling perspective, Super's theory offers several advantages over more traditional trait-and-factor approaches. For example, the developmental perspective of the theory is quite congruent with the progressive philosophy of rehabilitation. Moreover, in delineating stages and the developmental tasks associated with those stages, it offers the counsellor specific guidelines for when and how to intervene. This is true not only for clients whose vocational development is retarded, but also for clients who are adventitiously disabled and may have "regressed" to an earlier stage and need assistance in reintegrating their self-concepts and redirecting their vocational activities.

It should also be observed that Super was the first vocational development theorist to identify similarities and differences between the career development of precareer vs. midcareer disabilities (Super, 1957). Specifically, Super believed that the midcareer disability would present special problems due to the necessity of the individual to reintegrate a modified self-concept. Two other concepts introduced by Super which are especially relevant for rehabilitation counsellors are the terms *multipotentiality* and *planfulness*. It was Super's contention that individuals are multipotential in terms of their potential vocational activities. This concept is particularly important for rehabilitation counsellors to keep in mind so that they do not "pigeon-hole" their clients into a specific occupation due to the client's disability. The concept of developing a sense of planfulness in clients is also an important goal for rehabilitation counsellors since many rehabilitation clients attribute to chance an inordinate amount of importance insofar as their futures are concerned.

Another prominent developmental theory is the one originally proposed by Ginzberg, Ginsburg, Axelrad, and Herma (1951). This theory reflects the multidisciplinary efforts of an economist, a psychiatrist-psychoanalyst, a sociologist, and a psychologist-psychoanalyst to develop and test a theory of occupational choice. It is generally regarded as the first attempt to explain occupational choice from a developmental perspective. Some of the key elements of the theory are the following:

1. Occupational choice is a developmental process. Although the Ginzberg theory was later revised to view this process as lifelong, emphasis has always remained on the years from childhood to early adulthood (Ginzberg, 1972);
2. The developmental process is irreversible (i.e., the individual cannot return psychologically, physically, socially, etc., to the point where earlier decisions could be repeated). This aspect of the original theory was severely criticized and later was modified by Ginzberg (1972). Essentially, the term optimization was substituted for the term irreversibility. Specifically, it was concluded that the individual would optimize on those personal, economic, and social factors which influence a vocational decision at any particular time (Osipow, 1983);
3. There are three major periods and several substages. These periods and substages are as follows:
   Periods
   I. Fantasy period
   II. Tentative period (ages 11-18)
      1. Interest
      2. Capacity
      3. Values
      4. Transition
         III. Realistic Period (ages 18-24)
         1. Exploration
         2. Crystallization
         3. Specification
   Research suggests that the periods and substages exist pretty much as presented in the theory but that they probably occur earlier than hypothesized;
4. The four most important variables involved in occupational choice are (a) the reality factor, (b) the educational process, (c) emotional factors, and (d) individual values. Related to these four variables are the following critical developmental tasks: (a) reality testing, (b) the development of a suitable

time perspective, (c) the ability to defer gratification, and (d) the ability to accept and implement compromise.

In developing their theory, Ginzberg and his associates borrowed significantly from psychoanalysis, not only in terms of the importance accorded to the reality factor and the role of emotional factors, but also in terms of their classification of persons into two basic types: work-oriented persons and pleasure-oriented persons. They also recognized the importance of identification in the choice process and basically described people as being either active or passive.

While research support for the Ginzberg theory is sparse at best, there is, as noted previously, some support for the sequencing of the developmental periods. Also significant is the role which the theory played in stimulating others to examine more systematically the occupational choice process as well as the introduction of a developmental perspective.

In terms of practical application in rehabilitation settings, the theory's strongest asset is the presentation of a model that can be used to assist clients in moving from one developmental period to another. This aspect of the theory may be especially useful to counsellors who work with at-risk adolescents and other populations whose vocational development has been retarded by cognitive, physical, or social factors. Specifically, the counsellor can help the client move from one stage to another (e.g., capacity to values) by structuring activities which will help the individual to clarify those attributes or complete those tasks which are associated with a particular stage. The counsellor can also attempt to instill in the client those attributes which Ginzberg and his associates have identified as critical ingredients to making adequate vocational choices, namely, reality testing, the development of a suitable time perspective, the ability to defer gratification, and the ability to accept and implement compromises.

In addition to Super's theory and the theory presented by Ginzberg and his associates, another developmental theory which has had considerable impact was developed by Tiedeman and O'Hara (1963). This theory has since been refined and adapted to a variety of situations in a series of books and articles by Tiedeman and his associates (Dudley and Tiedeman, 1977; Miller-Tiedeman and Tiedeman, 1982; Tiedeman, 1979). In the

Tiedeman theory, emphasis is placed especially on the process of vocational decision-making, which is essentially characterized as having two major phases: anticipation and implementation. The anticipation phase includes the following aspects -- exploration, crystallization, choice, and clarification. The implementation phase includes induction, reaffirmation, and integration.

Like Super, Tiedeman places considerable importance on self development, which he believes proceeds as the result of ego-relevant crises. This aspect of this theory is closely tied to Erikson's (1959; 1963) eight psychosocial crises: (a) trust, (b) autonomy, (c) initiative, (d) industry, (e) identity, (f) intimacy, (g) generativity and (h) ego integrity. It is Tiedeman's belief that as one resolves these psychosocial crises, the person's ego identity develops and as a result, the person is better able to make well-informed career decisions.

Two other concepts which are critically important to Tiedeman's theory are *differentiation* and *integration*. Differentiation of the self is a complex and ongoing process which is influenced by biological, psychological, social, and situational factors. In vocational terms it is the person's view of the self in relation to various occupations and work activities. The manner in which one changes the work environment to fit the self and changes the self to fit the work environment constitutes the process of *integration*. Osipow (1983, p. 209) summarizes the major notions of career decision-making, as embodied in the Tiedeman theory, as follows:

1. Career development is built on ego identity continuously differentiating based on experience;
2. Among the ways this differentiating begins include the individual's problem solving set; and
3. This "condition of rational differentiation is important because (a) it represents a higher-level form of differentiation and (b) its rationability forms the basis on which counselling and guidance practices are designed."

While the vocational decision-making paradigm presented by Tiedeman and his associates has the advantage of emphasizing the cognitive and problem-solving aspects of career development, the theory is somewhat less than a panacea. It is a difficult theory to understand and does not have a substantial research basis. It does, however, offer the advantage of comprehensiveness and a specific focus on the vocational-choice process, which it proposes will recur each time the individual is required or decides to alter his/her career. This latter feature of the theory could be especially useful to rehabilitation counsellors who might use the various aspects of anticipation and implementation to help clients who are adventitiously or congenitally disabled to approach their career choices systematically. Another aspect of the theory, borrowed from Erikson (1959; 1963), which could be useful is the idea that growth and identity result primarily from crisis. This point of view could be helpful to counsellor and client alike when considering the potentially positive long-term effects of disability.

Rehabilitation Theories

Two theories of vocational behaviour which are particularly relevant to rehabilitation counselling are the Minnesota Theory of Work Adjustment (Dawis, 1967; Dawis, England, and Lofquist, 1964; Dawis and Lofquist, 1976; 1984; Dawis, Lofquist, and Weiss, 1968; Lofquist and Dawis, 1969; 1972; 1978) and McMahon's Model of Vocational Redevelopment (McMahon 1977, 1979). The first of these theories focusses on the concept of work adjustment in general, and the second on the vocational redevelopment of persons with a midcareer physical disability.

The Minnesota Theory of Work Adjustment is, in the Minnesota tradition, based on a trait-and-factor perspective of counselling. It was developed and validated over a period of several years at the University of Minnesota under the auspices of the "Minnesota Studies in Vocational Rehabilitation - Work Adjustment Project". Lofquist, Dawis, and their associates have authored numerous research monographs, articles, books, and chapters which describe the development, validation, and application of the theory.

The Minnesota Theory of Work Adjustment is based essentially on the concept of correspondence between the individual and the work environment. Specifically, the term *correspondence* is used to refer to the degree to which the individual fulfills the requirements of the work environment as well as the degree to which the work environment fulfills the requirements of the individual. The process by which the individual seeks to achieve and maintain correspondence is called *work adjustment* (hence, the name of the theory), and the stability of this work adjustment is referred to as *tenure on the job*. Two other terms which are particularly important in this theoretical model are *satisfaction* and *satisfactoriness*. The term *satisfaction* refers to the extent to which the work environment fulfills the requirements of the individual. In other words, to what extent does the reinforcer system of the work environment (i.e., working conditions, prestige, compensation, etc.) meet the needs of the individual (i.e., ability utilization, activity, security, social status, etc.)? *Satisfactoriness*, on the other hand, refers to the extent to which the abilities of the individual (i.e., general intelligence, mechanical ability, dexterity, etc.) meet the demands of the work environment. When considered jointly, these two concepts, satisfaction and satisfactoriness, indicate the degree of correspondence between the individual and the work environment and can be used to predict job tenure.

An advantage of the Minnesota Theory of Work Adjustment over most other vocational theories is that terms such as satisfaction, satisfactoriness, needs, abilities, ability requirements, and reinforcer systems have been operationally defined, and specific psychometric instruments have been developed by Lofquist, Dawis, and others to measure them. Among these instruments are the Minnesota Satisfaction Questionnaire (MSQ), Minnesota Satisfactoriness Scales (MSS), Minnesota Importance Questionnaire (MIQ), and Occupational Reinforcer Patterns (ORP). In addition, a variety of other psychometric instruments and related techniques (e.g., work samples, job analysis, and job tryouts) are available to assist counsellors to assess client abilities and needs and job demands and reinforcers.

Like other trait-and-factor approaches, the Minnesota Theory of Work Adjustment suffers from at least two major drawbacks: (a) Counsellors may not always assume that the psychometric and other techniques available to implement the theory will be reliable and valid for the specific individual and work environment in question; and (b) counsellors must not assume that the individual and work environments assessed will not change significantly in the future. If these limitations are kept in mind, the Minnesota Theory of Work Adjustment can provide the counsellor with a highly useful model from which to view and facilitate vocational decision-making and work adjustment.

In terms of rehabilitation counselling, perhaps the most relevant "developmental" theory was presented by Brian T. McMahon (1977, 1979). While McMahon's theory, called the Model of Vocational Redevelopment, is really more of a trait-and-factor theory than a developmental theory, it does address an issue of primary concern to many rehabilitation counsellors. Specifically, what factors are involved in the vocational redevelopment of persons with physical disabilities who are in mid-career?

McMahon's model, which he developed when he was a Ph.D. student at the University of Wisconsin-Madison, is based in part on previous efforts by Lofquist and Dawis (1969, 1972) and Hershenson (1974) to explain the work adjustment and vocational development of persons with a disability. It is in this sense that McMahon describes his model as being evolutionary rather than revolutionary.

McMahon (1977, 1979) proposed that work adjustment is essentially a goodness-of-fit between commensurate sets of worker dimensions and job dimensions. The worker dimensions include worker needs (e.g., advancement, security, social status, etc.) and worker competencies (worker abilities and worker adaptive abilities). The job dimensions include job reinforcer and job demands. Both the worker dimensions and the job dimensions are assumed to have subjective and objective components (i.e., what workers really need versus what they think they need, what is actually required for successful job performance versus what is thought to be required, etc.). McMahon believed that by assessing these various dimensions, the counsellor can provide estimates of worker-job fit, the accuracy of the worker's self assessment and the accuracy of the worker's self understanding. In addition, McMahon takes the very controversial position that a disability in mid-career is only important in terms of vocational development to the extent that it alters the needs or competencies of the worker or the reinforcers or demands of the job.

Two advantages of the McMahon model over other theories are:

1. It was developed specifically to explain and predict the vocational redevelopment of persons with a disability in mid-career; and
2. It encourages the counsellor to focus on factors which are directly related to work adjustment.

The model does, however, have several disadvantages. Among these are the following:

1. There has been no attempt by McMahon to validate or extend his work empirically;
2. The theory could probably be more aptly called a work readjustment or job placement theory than a vocational redevelopment theory, since there is really no attempt to describe the vocational redevelopment process *per se* (i.e., what are the stages and tasks involved in vocational redevelopment?);
3. Little is offered in terms of specific recommendations on how to use the theory;
4. The model places virtually no emphasis on extra-vocational factors such as the family or robustness of the economy, nor on factors such as the type, severity, or duration of the disability.

McMahon's theory provides a useful model for identifying essential factors in the return-to-work process (i.e., worker needs and competencies and job reinforcers and requirements); however, it falls short in terms of explaining the process of vocational redevelopment. It has also failed to command the attention and interest of the research community in rehabilitation counselling. This neglect is truly unfortunate since the theory represents a creative adaptation and extension of the Minnesota Theory of Work Adjustment and could be expanded to explain work adjustment processes in people who become disabled in pre-career or mid-career.

SUMMARY AND RECOMMENDATIONS

Selected theories of counselling and psychotherapy and career development and occupational choice are reviewed and critiqued in this chapter. Each theory is discussed in terms of its applicability to rehabilitation settings and clients. In addition, a model is provided which rehabilitation practitioners can use to evaluate the appropriateness of specific theories for use in their everyday practice. Presented below is a list of major ideas and recommendations:

1. Rehabilitation interventions are much too complex to be applied randomly. Thus, it is critically important that rehabilitation practice be derived from theory;
2. The practitioner's evaluations of a specific theory should include the following components:
   (a) whether the theory is congruent with the practitioner's basic philosophy and theoretical orientation;
   (b) whether the theory is well-developed, generalizable, and verifiable;
   (c) whether the theory is amenable to the measurement of change in the client's behaviour;
   (d) whether the theory is congruent with the practitioner's training and personality characteristics;
   (e) whether the theory is applicable to the specific clients served by the practitioner; and
   (f) whether the theory can be directed to goals acceptable to the counsellor, client, and work setting;
3. Psychodynamic theories of counselling and psychotherapy offer the practitioner a framework for understanding the structure of personality, the role of the unconscious and intrapsychic conflict, and the mechanisms of defense as these relate to rehabilitation and disability processes;
4. Humanistic theories provide the practitioner with critical information on the characteristics of the helping relationship and the importance of client-centred interventions;
5. Cognitive theories offer the practitioner systematic methods and instruments to assist clients in vocational and

educational decision-making and in improving social skills and self-esteem;

6. Behavioural approaches provide concrete and systematic methods for assisting clients in decision-making, reducing undesirable behaviour, increasing productivity, reducing anxiety and improving social skills and self-esteem;

7. Personality-based career development and occupational choice theories provide a structure for classifying occupations and a means for relating the personality characteristics of clients to that structure;

8. Developmental vocational theories offer the practitioner a framework from which to view career development and vocational decision-making in terms of developmental periods and stages. Such a framework is useful to practitioners in directing their interventions for clients with disabilities first occurring in pre or mid-career;

9. And finally, practitioners can use McMahon's Model of Vocational Redevelopment and the Minnesota Theory of Work Adjustment to direct their vocational assessment and job-placement functions in a variety of rehabilitation contexts.

REFERENCES

Bergin, A.F. and Garfield, S.L. (1971) *Handbook of Psychotherapy and Behavior Change*, John Wiley, New York.

Breuer, J. and Freud, S., (1893-1895) 'Studies in Hysteria', in J. Strachey (ed and trans), *The Standard Edition of the Complete Psychological Works of Sigmund Freud* (vol.2). Hogarth Press, London, 1955.

Brown, D. and Brooks, L. and Associates (1984) *Career Choice and Development*, Jossey-Bass, Inc., San Francisco.

Buehler, C. (1933) *Der Menschiliche Lebenslauf als Psychologiches Problem*, Hirzel, Leipzig.

Carkhuff, R.R. and Berenson, B.G. (1977) *Beyond Counselling and Therapy* (2nd ed), Holt, Rinehart and Winston, New York.

Cook, D. (1987) 'Psychosocial Impact of Disability', in R.M. Parker (ed), *Rehabilitation Counseling: Basics and Beyond*, Pro-Ed, Austin, Texas.

Corsini, R.J. (ed) (1981) *Handbook of Innovative Psychotherapies*, John Wiley, New York.

Cubbage, M.E. and Thomas, K.R. (1989) 'Freud and Disability', *Rehabilitation Psychology*, 34, 161-173.

Dawis, R.V. (1967) 'The Minnesota Studies in Vocational Rehabilitation', *Rehabilitation Counseling Bulletin*, 11, 1-10.

Dawis, R.V., England, G.W. and Lofquist, L.H. (1964) 'A Theory of Work Adjustment', *Minnesota Studies in Vocational Rehabilitation*, *XV*, University of Minnesota Industrial Relations Center, Minneapolis.

Dawis, R.V. and Lofquist, L.H. (1976) 'Personality Style and the Process of Work Adjustment', *Journal of Counseling Psychology*, 23, 55-59.

Dawis, R.V. and Lofquist, L.H. (1984) *A Psychological Theory of Work Adjustment: An Individual Differences Model and its Applications*, University of Minnesota Press, Minneapolis.

Dawis, R.V., Lofquist, L.H. and Weiss, D.J. (1968) 'A Theory of Work Adjustment: A Revision', *Minnesota Studies in Vocational Rehabilitation*, *XXIII*, University of Minnesota Industrial Relations Center, Minneapolis.

Dollard, J. and Miller, N.E. (1950) *Personality and Psychotherapy*, McGraw-Hill, New York.

Dudley, G.A. and Tiedeman, D.V. (1977) *Career Development: Exploration and Commitment*, Accelerated Development, Muncie, IN.

Ellis, A. (1960) *Reason and Emotion in Psychotherapy*, Lyle Stewart, New York.

Ellis, A. (1984) 'Rational-emotive Therapy', in R. Corsini (ed), *Current Psychotherapies* (3rd ed.), F.E. Peacock, Itasca, Il.

Erickson, E.H. (1959) 'Identity and the Life Cycle', *Psychological Issues*, 1.

Erickson, E.H. (1963) *Childhood and Society* (2nd ed.), Norton, New York.

Freud, A. (1936) *The Ego and the Mechanisms of Defense*, International Universities Press, New York.

Freud, S. (1923) 'The Ego and the Id', in J. Strachey (ed and trans), *The Standard Edition of the Complete Psychological Works of Sigmund Freud*, Hogarth Press, London, 1961, (Vol. 19).

Ginzberg, E. (1952) 'Toward a Theory of Occupational Choice', *Occupations*, 30, 491-494.

Ginzberg, E. (1970) 'The Development of a Developmental Theory of Occupational Choice', in W.H. Van Hoose and J.J. Pietrofesa (eds), *Counselling and Guidance in the Twentieth Century*, Houghton Mifflin, Boston.

Ginzberg, E. (1972) 'Toward a Theory of Occupational Choice: A Restatement', *Vocational Guidance Quarterly, 20,* 169- 176.

Ginzberg, E. (1984) 'Career Development', in D. Brown, L. Brooks and Associates (eds), *Career Choice and Development,* Jossey-Bass, Inc., San Francisco.

Ginzberg, E., Ginsburg, S.W., Axelrad, S. and Herma, J.L. (1951) *Occupational Choice: An Approach to a General Theory,* Columbia University Press, New York.

Glasser, W. (1965) *Reality Therapy,* Harper and Row, New York.

Glasser, W. (1969) *Schools Without Failure,* Harper and Row, New York.

Glasser, W. (1984) 'Reality Therapy', in R. Corsini (ed), *Current Psychotherapies,* F.E. Peacock, Itasca, Il.

Gottfriedson, G., Holland, J. and Ogawa, D. (1982) *Dictionary of Holland Occupational Codes,* Consulting Psychologists Press, Palo Alto, CA.

Hershenson, D.B. (1974) 'Vocational Guidance and the Handicapped', in E.L. Herr (ed), *Vocational Guidance and Human Development,* Houghton Mifflin, Boston.

Holland, J. (1966) *The Psychology of Vocational Choice: A Theory of Personality Types and Model Environments,* Blaisdell, Waltham, MA.

Holland, J. (1973) *Making Vocational Choices: A Theory of Careers,* Prentice-Hall, Englewood Cliffs, NJ.

Holland, J. (1985a) *Making Vocational Choices: A Theory of Vocational Personalities and Work Environments* (2nd ed.), Prentice Hall, Englewood Cliffs, NJ.

Holland, J. (1985b) *The Self-Directed Search: Professional Manual - 1985 edition,* Psychological Assessment Resources, Odessa, FL.

Hosford, R.E. and deVisser, L.A. (1974) *Behavioral Approaches to Counseling: An Introduction,* American Personnel and Guidance Association Press, Washington, DC.

Isaacson, L. (1985) *Basics of Career Counseling,* Allyn and Bacon, Boston.

Kempler, W. (1973) 'Gestalt Therapy', in R. Corsini (ed), *Current Psychotherapies* (2nd ed), F.E. Peacock, Itasca, IL.

Kiesler, D.J. (1973) *The Process of Psychotherapy,* Aldine, Chicago.

Kohut, H. (1984) *How Does Analysis Cure?,* University of Chicago Press, Chicago.

Krueger, D.W. (1984) 'Psychological Rehabilitation of Physical Trauma and Disability', in D.W. Krueger (ed), *Rehabilitation*

Psychology: A Comprehensive Textbook, Aspen, Rockville, MD.

Krumboltz, J. (1966) 'Behavioral Goals of Counseling', *Journal of Counseling Psychology, 13*, 153- 159.

Krumboltz, J. and Thoreson, C.E. (eds), (1969) *Behavioral Counseling: Cases and Techniques*, Holt, New York.

Krumboltz, J. and Thoreson, C.E. (eds), (1976) *Counseling Methods*, Holt, New York.

Levitsky, A. and Perls, F.S. (1970) 'The Rules and Games of Gestalt Therapy', in J. Fagan and I. Shepherd (eds), *Gestalt Therapy Now*, Science and Behavior Books, Palo Alto, CA.

Lewin, K. (1951) *Field Theory in Social Science*, University of Chicago Press, Chicago.

Lofquist, L.H. and Dawis, R.V. (1969) *Adjustment to Work: A Psychosocial View of Man's Problems in a Work-Oriented Society*, Appleton Century-Crofts, New York.

Lofquist, L.H. and Dawis, R.V. (1972) 'Application of the Theory of Work Adjustment to Rehabilitation and Counseling', *Minnesota Studies in Vocational Rehabilitation, XLVIII*, University of Minnesota Industrial Relations Center, Minneapolis.

Lofquist, L.H. and Dawis, R.V. (1978) 'Values as Secondary to Needs in the Theory of Work Adjustment,' *Journal of Vocational Behaviour, 12*, 12- 19.

Maslow, A. (1954) *Motivation and Personality*, Harper and Row, New York.

Meador, B. and Rogers, C. (1984) 'Person-centered Therapy', in R. Corsini (ed), *Current Psychotherapies* (3rd ed.), F.E. Peacock, Itasca, Il.

McMahon, B.T. (1977) A Model of Vocational Redevelopment for the Mid-Career Physically Disabled, unpublished Doctoral Dissertation, University of Wisconsin-Madison.

McMahon, B.T. (1979) 'A Model of Vocational Redevelopment for the Midcareer Physically Disabled', *Rehabilitation Counseling Bulletin, 23*, 35- 47.

Miller-Tiedeman, A.L. and Tiedeman, D.V. (1982) *Career Development: Journey into Personal Power*, Character Research Press, Schenectady, NY.

National Occupational Information Coordinating Committee, U.S. Department of Labor, (1986) *Using Labor Market Information in Career Exploration*, Garrett Park Press, Garrett Park, Md.

Neff, W.S. (1985) *Work and Human Behavior* (3rd ed), Aldine, New York.

O'Hara, R.P. and Tiedeman, D.V. (1959) 'Vocational Self Concept in Adolescents', *Journal of Counseling Psychology, 6*, 292- 301.

Osipow, S.H. (1983) *Theories of Career Development* (3rd ed), Prentice Hall, Inc., Englewood Cliffs, N.J.

Passons, W.R. (1975) *Gestalt Approaches in Counseling*, Holt, Rinehart and Winston, New York.

Patterson, C.H. (1986) *Theories of Counseling and Psychotherapy* (4th ed), Harper and Row, New York.

Perls, F. (1969) *Gestalt Therapy Verbatim*, Real People Press, Lafayette, CA.

Perls, F., Hefferline, R.F. and Goodman, P. (1951) *Gestalt Therapy*, Julian Press, New York.

Polster, E. and Polster, M. (1973) *Gestalt Therapy Integrated*, Brunner/Mazel, New York.

Roe, A. (1956) *The Psychology of Occupations*, John Wiley and Sons, New York.

Rogers, C.R. (1942) *Counseling and Psychotherapy*, Houghton Mifflin, Boston.

Rogers, C.R. (1951) *Client-Centered Therapy*, Houghton Mifflin, Boston.

Rogers, C.R. (1961) *On Becoming a Person: A Therapist's View of Psychotherapy*, Houghton Mifflin, Boston.

Rogers, C.R., Gendlin, E.T., Kiesler, D.J. and Truax, C.B. (eds) (1967) *The Therapeutic Relationship and its Impact: A Study of Psychotherapy with Schizophrenics*, The University of Wisconsin Press, Madison, WI.

Shorkey, C. and Whiteman, V. (1977) 'Development of the Rational Behavior Inventory', *Educational and Psychological Measurement, 37*, 527- 534.

Siller, J. (1988) 'Intrapsychic Aspects of Attitudes Toward Persons with Disabilities', in H.E. Yuker (ed), *Attitudes Toward Persons with Disabilities*, Springer, New York. (pp. 58- 67).

Simkin, J. and Yontif, G. (1984) 'Gestalt Therapy', in R. Corsini (ed), *Current Psychotherapies* (3rd ed), F.E. Peacock, Itasca, Il.

Snygg, D. and Combs, A.W. (1949) *Individual Behavior*, Harper and Row, New York.

Super, D.E. (1953) 'A Theory of Vocational Development', *American Psychologist, 8*, 185-190.

Super, D.E. (1957) *The Psychology of Careers: An Introduction to Career Development*, Harper and Row, New York.

Super, D.E. (1964) 'A Developmental Approach to Vocational Guidance', *Vocational Guidance Quarterly, 13*, 1- 10.

Super, D.E. (1969) 'Vocational Development Theory', *The Counselling Psychologist, 1*, 2 -30.

Super, D.E. (1980) 'A Life-span, Life-space, Approach to Career Development', *Journal of Vocational Behaviour, 16*, 284-298.

Super, D.E. (1984) 'Career and Life Development', in D. Brown, L. Brooks and Associates (eds), *Career Choice and Development*, Jossey-Bass, Inc., San Francisco.

Super, D.E. and Bachrach, P. (1957) *Scientific Careers and Vocational Development Theory*, Teachers College Press, New York.

Thomas, K.R., Butler, A.J. and Parker, R.M. (1987) 'Psychosocial Counseling', in R.M. Parker (ed), *Rehabilitation Counseling: Basics and Beyond*, Pro-Ed, Austin, TX.

Thomas, K.R. and McGinnis, J.D. (in press) 'The Psychoanalytic Theories of D.W. Winnicott as Applied to Rehabilitation', *Journal of Rehabilitation*.

Tiedeman, D.V. (1961) 'Decisions and Vocational Development: A Paradigm and its Implications', *Personnel and Guidance Journal, 40*, 15- 21.

Tiedeman, D.V. (1979) *Career Development: Designing our Career Machines*, Character Research Press, Schenectady, NY.

Tiedeman, D.V. and Miller-Tiedeman, A. (1979) 'Choice and Decision Processes and Career Revisited', in A.M. Mitchell, G. B. Jones, and J.D. Krumboltz (eds), *Social Learning and Career Decision Making*, Carroll Press, Cranston, RI.

Tiedeman, D.V. and Miller-Tiedeman, A. (1984) 'Career Decision Making: An Individualistic Perspective', in D. Brown, L. Brooks and Associates (eds), *Career Choice and Development*, Jossey-Bass, Inc., San Francisco.

Tiedeman, D.V. and O'Hara, R.P. (1963) *Career Development: Choice and Adjustment*, College Entrance Examination Board, New York.

Williamson, E.G. (1950) *Counseling Adolescents*, McGraw-Hill, New York.

Williamson, E.G. (1965) *Vocational Counseling*, McGraw-Hill, New York.

Winnicott, D.W. (1975) *Through Paediatrics to Psycho-analysis*, Basic Books, Inc., New York.

Wolpe, J. (1958) *Psychotherapy by Reciprocal Inhibition*, Stanford University Press, Stanford, CA.

Wolpe, J. (1969) *The Practice of Behavior Therapy*, Pergamon, New York.

Zunker, V. (1986) *Career Counseling: Applied Concepts of Life Planning* (2nd ed), Brooks/Cole, Monterey, CA.

Chapter Four

A COGNITIVE APPROACH TO COUNSELLING CLIENTS WITH PHYSICAL DISABILITIES

James W. Vargo

INTRODUCTION

Adjustment to disability is a complex phenomenon that is affected by many factors (Livneh, 1986; Vargo, 1978; Vash, 1981; Wright, 1983). One of the most compelling of these is attitudes: attitudes of the general public, of rehabilitation and other health professionals, and of people with disabilities themselves. Because individuals with disabilities are indoctrinated by the same attitudes, prejudices, and stereotypes as mainstream society, many of the hurdles they encounter on the road to adjustment are products of cognitions and self-verbalizations. As a result, cognitive approaches to counselling and psychotherapy provide powerful methods of overcoming dysfunctional behaviour patterns, thereby releasing clients to more productive, satisfying lives.

This chapter briefly overviews some of the attitudinal factors affecting adjustment, presents the core components of cognitive-behavioural approaches to counselling and therapy, and reviews the literature on the application of cognitive-behavioural methods to clients with disabilities. The chapter concludes by identifying ten self-defeating thoughts common to persons with disabilities and recommending specific techniques for helping clients to overcome them.

ATTITUDES AND ADJUSTMENT

Attitudes of the general public toward people with physical disabilities are a potent influence on rehabilitation and adjustment (Roeher, 1961) and much of the research in this area suggests that these attitudes are, for the most part, negative (For reviews and analyses of this literature, see Marinelli and Dell Orto, 1977; Vargo, 1985; Westwood, Vargo and Vargo, 1981; Wetstein-Kroft and Vargo, 1984; Wright, 1983.) In fact, negative attitudes are so prevalent that one book on the subject is entitled *Disabled People as Second-Class Citizens* (Eisenberg, Griggins and Duval, 1982). In the introduction to that work, Eisenberg states:

> [Living with a disability] often means living at the poverty level and going on welfare. It means *discrimination* (original emphasis). Being disabled is not just having a body defect – it is a complex social-political reality that one lives with day by day, year by year (Eisenberg, 1982, p. xiv).

Beatrice Wright (1983), a major writer in this area, has classified unrealistic attitudes toward people with disabilities in terms of two "status positions": inferior status and salutary status. Persons with disabilities relegated by others to the inferior status position are generally viewed as being less worthwhile than other people on dimensions other than those circumscribed by the disability itself. The salutary status position, on the other hand, reflects the view that people with disabilities are supernormal in that they are more courageous, kinder, more sensitive, and the like than are people without disabilities. These two positions are not mutually exclusive; the status granted is usually situation dependent. These stereotypical attitudes toward people with disabilities are perpetuated by a number of means including literature, movies, and other media sources.

Thurer (1980) argues that physical disability, as portrayed in art and literature, is nearly always wrapped in metaphor, usually as a symbol of what Thurer terms "monstrosity". Weinberg and Santana (1978) rated 63 physically deformed comic book characters according to whether they were portrayed as being morally evil, good, or neutral. Their results indicated that 57% were presented as being evil, 43% as good, and 0% as neutral. Thus there were no "ordinary" characters. Results are similar for movies. In their review of over 1,000 feature films,

Byrd and Elliott (1985) found 120 which depicted someone with a disability. Of these, 98 were judged to be negative and 22 positive.

Fund-raising campaigns also frequently impart messages which equate disability with suffering and tragedy (Wright, 1983). Too often these campaigns appeal to pity and guilt in an attempt to loosen the public's purse-strings. The point is that rarely do the media present people with disabilities as ordinary people who happen to have a physical problem.

Physical disability is often an assault on one's self concept. Adjustment means not only learning how to best manage one's physical environment, but also developing a new self concept, one that is cemented in different values regarding what it means to be worthwhile. It should come as no surprise, therefore, that this fragile period of redevelopment is strongly influenced by the attitudes and reactions of those people who spend the most time in the company of the person with the disability, namely rehabilitation professionals. McDaniel (1976) has argued that attitudes of health professionals are probably more important than any other factor in influencing the client's response to rehabilitation. And not all these attitudes are positive. For example, Crunk and Allen's (1977) investigation of five different groups of rehabilitation workers concluded that all had negative attitudes toward people with disabilities and that certain of the rehabilitation groups were more negative than others.

At first glance, it might appear that people with disabilities would have positive attitudes toward other people with disabilities. However, this is not usually the case. People with disabilities are members of a given culture just like anyone else and, as such, are prone to the same beliefs as mainstream society (Westwood *et al.*, 1981; Wetstein-Kroft and Vargo, 1984). It is clear that certain societies are better than others at accepting individuals who are visibly different (Jaques, Linkowski and Sieka, 1970; Schneider and Anderson, 1980; Westwood and Vargo, 1985) and this has a profound impact on individuals with disabilities' views of disability in general and their own specific situation in particular. Some societies and cultures place great emphasis on what I call the "ideology of normality". By this I mean that they promote the belief that to be "normal" is the highest value and any deviation from that society's definition of normality is intrinsically undesirable, and therefore to be avoided at all costs. Consequently, individuals with disabilities harbour many of the same myths and stereotypes about disability as everyone else because they are exposed to the same purveyors of attitudes. In her summary of the research on attitudes of persons with disabilities toward others with disability, Dixon (1977) concluded that people with disabilities do hold negative attitudes toward others with disabilities but that these attitudes are not as negative as those held by people who do not have disabilities. Furthermore, there is a tendency for people with disabilites to hold more favourable attitudes toward others with the same disability.

What this means in terms of personal adjustment to disability is that it is not only the sector of society that is free from disabilities which assimilates these stereotypical notions of what it means to have a disability. People with disabilities incorporate them as well, making it even more difficult to escape from the emotional chains which prevent or delay the adoption of values which are necessary for transition to a life of new perspectives. This is reflected in a study by Mayer and Eisenberg (1982) that found the self-concept scores of a group of spinal cord individuals to be lower than those of the general population and higher than those of a sample of psychiatric patients. Some writers (e.g., Kottke, 1982; Vargo, 1986) have argued that, because of the problems associated with living with a severe disability, a sound philosophy of life may be even more important for people who have disabilities than for those who don't. It is the development of this "sound philosophy of life" that forms the basis of the cognitive-behavioural movement in psychology and psychotherapy.

COGNITIVE BEHAVIOUR THERAPY

Cognitive behaviour therapy (CBT) was originally developed as an extension of behaviour therapy. Nearly all forms of behaviour therapy are stimulus-response approaches while CBT takes the extra step of recognizing the importance of thought (cognition) as a psychological filter which mediates between stimulus and response.

All forms of Cognitive Behaviour Therapy have a number of characteristics in common. CBT is an educational model of counselling and psychotherapy. Therapy is short-term, didactic, and directive. The basic premises underlying all forms of CBT are that:

1. Thoughts affect feelings;
2. One can alter one's feelings by thinking different thoughts. These premises are reflected in what Raimy (1975) calls the "Misconception Hypothesis":

> If those ideas or conceptions of a client or patient which are relevant to his psychological problems can be changed in the direction of greater accuracy where his reality is concerned, his maladjustments are likely to be eliminated. (p. 7)

The premises underlying CBT have been empirically validated. A variety of studies (e.g., Goldfried, Decenteceo, and Weinberg, 1974; Wickless and Kirsch, 1988) have clearly demonstrated that the way one views a situation has a powerful influence on how one reacts to it.

The cognitive-behavioural approach has become one of the major trends in counselling and psychotherapy in recent years, particularly in North America. Smith (1982) asked 800 members of the American Psychological Association to rank order the psychotherapists whom they considered to be the most influential today. Out of the ten top ranked therapists, four are identified with the cognitive-behavioural approach, more than for any other theoretical position. (Note: For the purposes of this discussion I am classifying rational-emotive therapy [RET] as a cognitive-behavioural approach since many authors [e.g., Ivey and Simek-Downing, 1987] consider Albert Ellis, the founder of RET, to be a pioneer of the cognitive-behavioural movement. However, it should be recognized that Ellis himself does distinguish between the two approaches [1980].)

In terms of the implementation of CBT, the following observations apply regardless of the specific form that is used (based on Wessler and Ellis, 1980):

1. The most effective practitioners of CBT tend to be therapists who already possess sound counselling skills;
2. The most difficult aspect of CBT is learning how to effectively

dispute the client's self-defeating thoughts;
3. CBT is often used in conjunction with other techniques such as relaxation training, behaviour rehearsal, and assertion training.

The application of CBT has been documented with such a diversity of conditions that it would be virtually impossible to document them all. A partial list includes borderline schizophrenia (Ellis, 1963), anxiety disorders and phobias (Beck, Emory and Greenberg, 1985), alcohol and substance abuse (Ellis, McInerney, DiGiuseppe, and Yeager, 1988), marital problems (Freeman, 1983), and everyday personal adjustment problems (Ellis, 1975; Ellis and Harper, 1975). In addition, a growing number of carefully controlled outcome studies have demonstrated the efficacy of CBT in the treatment of depression (e.g., Blackburn, Bishop, Glen, Whalley and Christie, 1981; Fuchs and Rehm, 1977; McLean and Hakstian, 1979; Rush, Beck, Kovacs and Hollon, 1977; Wilson, Goldin and Charbonneau-Powis, 1983). For further information regarding the practical application of Cognitive-Behavioural techniques, the reader is directed to a wide variety of handbooks in the area; e.g., Beck, 1976, 1988; Dobson, 1988; Ellis, 1962; Ellis and Bernard, 1985; Ellis and Grieger, 1977; Epstein, Schlesinger and Dryden, 1988; Foreyt and Rathjen, 1978; Freeman, 1983; and Meichenbaum, 1977.

COGNITIVE BEHAVIOUR THERAPY IN REHABILITATION

It has long been recognized that many individuals with physical disabilities experience emotional and behavioural problems which interfere with the adjustment process and that the difficulties in coming to terms with the disability are not a direct result of the physical constraints imposed by the disabling condition. For example, Ben-Sira (1981, 1983) has demonstrated that the degree of adjustment to disability is independent of the severity of the impairment. Why some persons adjust more quickly than others is, in large part, a function of self-verbalizations; that is, what they tell themselves about their disability. Despite the fact that such self-defeating verbalizations are prime candidates for Cognitive Behaviour Therapy, it is only recently that rehabilitation professionals have begun to employ cognitive-behavioural methods to help clients deal with adjustment problems.

The condition most often reported in the rehabilitation literature as having been treated with cognitive-behavioural techniques is chronic pain. A review and analysis of this literature is provided by Pearce (1983) who reports generally favourable results for cognitive methods in the management of chronic pain although she does caution that many of the studies are not well controlled.

One of the advantages of CBT is the ease with which it can be applied in group settings. This approach has been used to help individuals with a variety of conditions overcome depression and other negative emotions. Larcombe and Wilson (1984) treated two groups comprised of four and five individuals with multiple sclerosis with CBT for 1 1/2 hours per week over six weeks. When compared to ten patients on a waiting list control group, the treatment group showed significantly greater gains on four different measures of depression.

Davis, Armstrong, Donovan and Temkin (1984) compared eight patients with epilepsy who were treated with group CBT for two hours per week for six weeks with a control group of five patients. Participants in the treatment group demonstrated significant decreases on measures of depression, anger, and anxiety, and significant increases on measures of social activities.

Tarrier, Maguire and Kincey (1983) conducted a study which compared the use of CBT alone with CBT combined with medication using a group of mastectomy patients who were referred to a psychiatrist because of depression and poor adjustment to breast loss. At three month follow-up the women who had received medication in addition to CBT showed greater gains than the CBT alone group. However, these results must be viewed with considerable caution since at the time of follow-up there were only three women in each group.

An innovative application of CBT in rehabilitation is reported by Evans, Halar and Smith (1985). They randomly selected outpatients from a 16 bed rehabilitation centre and systematically assigned them to treatment (n=63) and control (n=64) groups. Outpatients in the treatment groups were exposed to cognitive-behavioural techniques via conference telephone calls. Sessions lasted one hour per week for eight weeks. Although pre-post test measures did not show significant differences between the treatment and control groups on indicators of depression and life satisfaction, the treatment groups did demonstrate less loneliness and more social skills than the control groups as a result of the telephone intervention.

Freeman and Greenwood (1987) have edited a text on cognitive therapy as applied to psychiatric and medical settings. Included are descriptions of CBT with patients who have cancer, head injuries, and those who exhibit Type A behaviour. Of particular relevance to this discussion is a chapter by Weinberg (1987) which addresses CBT applied to the sexual rehabilitation of individuals with spinal cord injuries. Weinberg provides a session-by-session outline of an eight-week group therapy programme designed to help spinal cord injured individuals come to terms with the sexual issues faced by all persons who acquire a disability through illness or injury.

Although some literature does claim to apply cognitive techniques to rehabilitation, with the exception of the Freeman and Greenwood text, there is very little which explicitly describes how cognitive-behavioural methods can be used with rehabilitation clients. For example, a paper by Ostby (1985), whose aim is to discuss rational-emotive therapy as a useful approach to rehabilitation counselling provides very little in the way of concrete techniques or examples that are specific to rehabilitation. A similar criticism applies to an article by Bowers (1988) entitled "Beck's Cognitive Therapy: An Overview for Rehabilitation Counsellors". Of the four journal pages occupied by the paper, only the last two paragraphs discuss implications for the rehabilitation counsellor. A somewhat better effort is provided by Gandy (1985) although here again no concrete techniques are offered. Therefore, the purpose of the remainder of this chapter is:

1. To identify self-defeating thoughts that are commonly held by people with disabilities; and
2. To propose cognitive-behavioural strategies for helping clients who have disabilities to dispute those thoughts and replace them with more productive ones.

I would like to caution at this point, however, that what follows may be applicable only to individuals with *acquired disabilities*. In all likelihood, people with congenital disabilities do not fit the pattern in the same way as those individuals who live a "normal" life during their primary years, then acquire a disability through illness or injury. Whether there is some critical period in life before which these observations do not apply is a question for future research to determine. In addition, let me caution that the cognitive-behavioural approach is not effective with individuals who exhibit loss of contact with reality as evidenced by symptoms such as delusions and hallucinations (e.g., major affective disorders, schizophrenic disorders and organic brain syndromes) or with clients who demonstrate impaired ability to reason and think logically (Beck, Rush and Shaw, 1979; Shaw, 1980).

SELF-DEFEATING THOUGHTS COMMON TO PERSONS WITH DISABILITIES

The previous caveats aside, I believe that psychological adjustment to disability is primarily a function of one's philosophy of life. It both determines, and is a reflection of, how one views what it means to be a person with a disability in terms of abilities, roles, and expectations. More specifically, it is one's cognitions that guide one's actions and reactions in life. Because of all the factors discussed previously, individuals with disabilities often harbour a number of cognitive distortions about themselves and their place in society. Such cognitive distortions have been called "mistaken beliefs" by Adler (Ansbacher and Ansbacher, 1956), "irrational ideas" by Ellis (1962), and "misconceptions" by Raimy (1975). A misconception is defined as a "faulty, mistaken, or erroneous conception" which fosters maladjustment (Raimy, 1975, p. 8). Personally I prefer the term "self-defeating thoughts" but feel equally comfortable with "misconceptions" and "irrational ideas".

Raimy (1975) has demonstrated that particular types of misconceptions may underlay specific psychiatric conditions and that these misconceptions seem to occur in clusters. Thus he has identified one cluster of misconceptions which are characteristic of depression, another which he calls "special person misconceptions", and so on. In a parallel fashion, I have proposed ten intrapersonal and interpersonal misconceptions or self-defeating thoughts which I believe are commonly held by people with disabilities (Vargo, 1989). The common feature of all these self-defeating thoughts is that they are a form of self-talk. They are as follows:

1. My disability is a punishment;
2. All of my difficulties are caused by my disability;
3. Asking for help is a sign of personal weakness;
4. I'm of less value as person because I'm not able-bodied;
5. It is impossible for a person with a disability to be happy;
6. No one can possibly understand how I feel;
7. I can't continue to live like this;
8. I can't do things the way I used to, so why do anything at all;
9. I can never succeed at anything;
10. Life can't possibly be fulfilling for me.

What makes individuals prone to such thoughts when they are so clearly self-defeating? Ellis (1976, 1979) has argued that all human beings seem to have a biological predisposition to indoctrinate themselves with irrational ideas, as Ellis calls them. Support for this contention has been provided in recent years by work which indicates that the bases for many human emotions are "hardwired" into our neurological structures (e.g., Greenberg and Safran, 1984, 1987; Safran and Greenberg, 1987). Emotionally-laden conceptions about the world are learned at an early age and it takes a concerted effort to overcome them, partly because much of their formation occurs at a subconscious (subcortical) level through the process of classical conditioning. Humans are social creatures with great needs for affection and affiliation, and this often means following the crowd regardless of how little justification there may be for what the crowd believes. Bertrand Russell once said that "if 50 million people say a foolish thing, it is still a foolish thing". Yet few people overcome the biological propensity to unquestioningly adopt all manner of foolishness and examine the empirical evidence for their beliefs.

In addition, everyone engages in self-talk and much of this self-talk is learned at an age when the individual is cognitively unequipped to examine it critically. Of course, this is what self-defeating thoughts are all about. They are self-statements that perpetuate unhealthy reactions to oneself and to others. And this is where I propose that counsellors direct their efforts: to assist clients in identifying, challenging, and disputing the self-defeating thoughts that form the basis of many of their difficulties. Each self-defeating thought (hereafter abbreviated as SDT) will be considered separately although it must be recognized that many of the suggested strategies are applicable to more than one particular SDT.

STRATEGIES FOR DISPUTING SELF-DEFEATING THOUGHTS

1. My disability is a punishment.

This SDT was identified by Wright (1983) as one of ten "hypotheses that support disability as a sign of personal inferiority" (p. 283). It is often accompanied by feelings of guilt, remorse and sinfulness. Overcoming these negative feelings requires changing the assumptions underlying the SDT. People with disabilities are more likely to reach a higher level of psychological health if they tell themselves that their disability is simply the result of an unfortunate accident or quirk of fate.

One technique that can be used is to ask: "Where is the proof?". However, counsellors must be rigorous about the type of evidence that is acceptable as proof. The point is, of course, that there is no 'proof' that disability is a punishment for real or imagined wrongdoings and it is imperative that the client come to realize that fact. This and other SDTs are often based on unexamined assumptions about how the world operates. Assumptions can be reevaluated in light of empirical evidence only when they are made explicit. Once this is done clients can be helped to reassess the empirical validity of their beliefs.

2. All of my difficulties are caused by my disabilities.

This SDT reflects the notion that all problems of individuals with disabilities are caused by the disability and, conversely, that if they did not have a disability they would not have problems. Of course, this isn't true. Everyone has problems, but it is important to help clients differentiate between those difficulties that are a result of the disability and those that are not. One of the challenges that clients must face is to learn to accept those aspects of their lives that can't be changed and to take a hard look at their own responsibility for life events before blaming everything on the disability. Some people with disabilities need help to assess their own personal strengths, then develop and nurture these to the point where disability recedes into the background and becomes a minor part of living.

Counsellors can help their clients discriminate between an event being bad or unpleasant versus it being awful or catastrophic. In part, this is a matter of reframing. For example, if a client believes that it is *unpleasant* or *inconvenient* to have to ride around in a wheelchair, then he or she will behave differently than if he or she believes that it is *horrible* or *catastrophic*. One can handle inconveniences much more easily than catastrophes.

3. Asking for help is a sign of personal weakness.

Many people who have disabilities must ask for help every day of their lives. They may have difficulty asking for help because we all learn at a very early age that our society equates dependence with inferiority. I'm sure that every person with a disability has experienced this difficulty from time to time. It can be unpleasant to request assistance when one would rather be independent - but does this make one less worthwhile as a human being? Of course not, yet this is a hard-earned lesson for many people to come by.

4. I'm of less value as a person because I'm not able-bodied.

This SDT was also reported by Wright (1983) as one of the beliefs that reflect the view that disability is a sign of personal inferiority. Disability can be a devastating experience for many people. In its initial stages, disability can shatter self-esteem. But some individuals continue to tell themselves that they are less worthwhile as human beings simply because they happen to have a disability. Clients need to realize that what makes people worthwhile has nothing to do with whether they have a disability or whether they are able-bodied; it has to do with their qualities as people and what they decide to do with their lives.

5. It is impossible for a person with a disability to be happy.

This SDT is a variation of the irrational belief that human unhappiness is caused by external events (Ellis, 1962), in this case, disability. In reality, however, persons' reactions to their disabilities are caused not by the physical limitations of the disabilities *per se* (Ben-Sira, 1981, 1983), but by what those individuals tell themselves about their disabilities - that they are awful, or terrible, or horrible, for instance. What is needed is first to get clients to identify and verbalize such self-statements, then to help them recognize that evaluations such as "awful", "terrible", and "horrible" are definitional labels that human beings attach to events. Nothing is intrinsically awful. Events just *are* and clients will save themselves much distress, suffering, and anger if they can adopt this philosophical position and get on with their lives, difficult though they may be.

6. No one can possibly understand how I feel.

This SDT usually has two components: a) It is impossible for anyone to understand what it means for me to live with my disability, and b) Other people *should* understand and accept me. Once the client has acknowledged these components, the following strategies may be appropriate. Each component is considered separately.

   (a) The first component is true only in so far as it is impossible for any one human being to understand the experience of any other. What clients usually really mean by this SDT is that it is impossible for anyone else to *experience* their disabilities and this, of course, is true. But that is quite a different matter from the abilities of a counsellor, or anyone else, to *understand* the position of a client who has a disability. Counsellors and many other health professionals, by virtue of their training and experience, have at their disposal a wide variety of techniques (e.g., paraphrasing, perception checking, and reflection) the very purpose of which is to facilitate understanding of the client's subjective experience. Use of these techniques may be the very thing that clients need to demonstrate to them that they are not alone and that someone (i.e., the counsellor) can and does understand them.

(b) The second component of this SDT is that other people (often this means everyone) should or must understand what it means to have a disability. Whenever such components as these emerge (Ellis calls them "musturbations"), it is useful for the counsellor to analyze and dispute the client's unrealistic "shoulds" since the word "should" has different connotations. When used as an indication of probability, "should" is appropriate (as in the statement, "If I mix blue and yellow, I should get green"). However if used to impose a *demand* on the world, it is inappropriate (as in "People should accept me just as I am"). The latter statement reflects a "should of obligation" as opposed to a "should of probability" (Vertes, 1971). It would be nice, desirable, and pleasant if people were totally accepting, but *should* they be?

7. I can't continue to live like this.

If this SDT is expressed, it is imperative that the counsellor quickly determine what is meant by it. If it is an expression of suicidal intention, for example, immediate action must be taken. However, in the majority of instances, such statements are not indications of death wishes or plans to take one's life but rather are further reflections of demandingness and awfulizing. In cases such as these, it is sometimes helpful to show the client who claims "I just can't stand it" that he or she *is* standing it; i.e., that although the client doesn't *like* it, he or she *is* enduring it. Awareness of this rather obvious fact can often be quite an eye-opener and usually leads to the more productive discussion of the distinction between "can't stand" versus "don't like" or "don't want to". The point is that all of us manage quite well in life while still engaging in activities that we don't like and would rather not do.

8. I can't do things the way I used to, so why do anything at all?

This SDT is a variation of the commonly held belief that life must always be fair to me. What most clients with disabilities are telling themselves in this instance is that *it's not fair* that they can no longer manage in the same way as they could before they acquired a disability and that *life should be fair*. This is often a difficult SDT to break but such clients need to come to realize that distress and unhappiness are caused in direct proportion to the extent that people demand that life must be fair. In reality, life pays no attention to one's demands; sometimes it is fair and sometimes it isn't.

9. I can never succeed at anything.

This SDT closely approximates to what Raimy (1985) refers to as "the incapacity misconception" - the unquestioned acceptance that one cannot engage in a certain activity or achieve a specified goal. With individuals whose disabilities are severe, this often generalizes to virtually *all* activities and goals.

Some clients can be helped by being shown that many of their current difficulties are logical outcomes of holding rigidly to their SDTs. For example, it is perfectly reasonable for clients who believe that they can never succeed to give up trying. Counsellors can point out to clients such as these that if other people held the same belief, they wouldn't try either. And, of course, not trying is the one way to guarantee that success will never come.

A variation of this SDT is often evident when a client claims that he or she can't engage in a certain activity that, in reality, is physically possible. A technique called "The Million Dollar Analogy" can be helpful here. An example of how it might be used is provided by the following exchange between a counsellor and a spinal cord injured client who refused to leave his home (Cl=Client; Co=Counsellor):

Cl: I just can't go out in public;
Co: You mean you won't;
Cl: No, I mean I can't. It's awful when people stare at you like you're some kind of creature from outer space;
Co: What if I gave you a million dollars to go out into public - then could you do it?;
Cl: (Laughs) You bet, for a million bucks I could;
Co: Then you *can* do it;
Cl: O.K., I could but I wouldn't like it.

10. Life can't possibly be fulfilling for me.

Contrary to this SDT, living with a disability can provide the opportunity to resolve issues in one's life that are less pressing for people who do not have disabilities. A disability forces people to face head-on many questions that other people do not consider until much later in life, for example, such issues as mortality, the meaning of life, and the relevance of physique and physical beauty to the concept of oneself as a worthwhile human being.

Many of the techniques discussed previously are useful for combating this SDT as well. Counsellors need to apply whatever strategies they have at their disposal to encourage clients to examine the validity of their self-defeating thoughts, particularly those that reflect components of demandingness and awfulizing (Bard, 1980; Ostby, 1985; Raimy, 1975; Wessler and Ellis, 1980).

RECOMMENDATIONS

1. If you are unfamiliar with CBT theory, read some of the handbooks referenced in this chapter.

2. Incorporate CBT techniques into your current counselling approach.

3. Use CBT in conjunction with other counselling methods that you already have some expertise with.

4. Select candidates for CBT carefully. They should be of average intelligence or better, verbally adept, and show no indications of brain damage or psychosis.

5. Assist the client in identifying the SDT that seems to be causing the most difficulties. Work on that one first.

6. Assign homework such as having the client identify and dispute SDTs as they occur.

7. Work on each emerging SDT in turn.

8. Assist the client in generalizing the progress made in

overcoming SDTs in one area to other areas of the client's life.

9. Help the client incorporate the benefits of CBT into an all-encompassing, productive philosophy of life.

A FINAL WORD

In conclusion, it is important for anyone considering the use of cognitive-behavioural methods to implement them only within a caring and supportive relationship. Clients respond to the techniques suggested in this chapter much better when they understand that it is their self-defeating thoughts that are being scrutinized, *not* the clients themselves. In addition, clients will understandably react defensively if they feel they are being attacked and judged as stupid or incompetent. Therefore, it is necessary for counsellors to utilize these techniques within a framework of advocacy and compassion. In that way, they can truly assist clients to forego demandingness and awfulizing in favour of a philosophical position that fosters self-acceptance and personal contentment.

REFERENCES

Ansbacher, H.L. and Ansbacher, R.R. (eds) (1956) *The Individual Psychology of Alfred Adler*, Harper and Row, New York.
Bard, J.A. (1980) *Rational Emotive Therapy in Practice*, Research Press, Champaign, IL.
Beck, A.T. (1976) *Cognitive Therapy and the Emotional Disorders*, International Universities Press, New York.
Beck, A.T. (1988) *Love is Never Enough*, Harper and Row, New York.
Beck, A.T., Emory, G. and Greenberg, R.L. (1985) *Anxiety Disorders and Phobias: A Cognitive Perspective*, Basic Books, New York.
Beck, A.T., Rush, A.J. and Shaw, B.F. (1979) *Cognitive Therapy of Depression*, Guilford, New York.
Ben-Sira, Z. (1981) 'The Structure of Readjustment of the Disabled: An Additional Perspective on Rehabilitation', *Social Science Medicine, 15A*, 565–581.

Ben Sira, Z. (1983) 'Loss, Stress and Readjustment: The Structure of Coping with Bereavement and Disability', *Social Science Medicine, 17,* 1619–1631.

Blackburn, I.M., Bishop, S., Glen, A.I.M., Whalley, L.J. and Christie, J.E. (1981) 'The Efficacy of Cognitive Therapy in Depression: A Treatment Trial Using Cognitive Therapy and Pharmacotherapy, Each Alone and in Combination', *British Journal of Psychiatry, 139,* 181–189.

Bowers, W.A. (1988) 'Beck's Cognitive Therapy: An Overview for Rehabilitation Counselors', *Journal of Applied Rehabilitation Counseling, 19(1),* 43–46.

Byrd, E.K. and Elliott, T.R. (1985) 'Feature Films and Disability: A Descriptive Study', *Rehabilitation Psychology, 30,* 47–51.

Crunk, W.A. Jr. and Allen, J. (1977) 'Attitudes Toward the Severely Disabled Among Five Rehabilitation Groups', *Journal of Applied Rehabilitation Counseling, 7(4),* 237–244.

Davis, G.R., Armstrong, H.E., Donovan, D.M. and Temkin, N.R. (1984) 'Cognitive-behavioral Treatment of Depressed Affect Among Epileptics: Preliminary Findings', *Journal of Clinical Psychology, 40,* 930–935.

Dixon, J.K. (1977) 'Coping with Prejudice: Attitudes of Handicapped Persons Toward the Handicapped', *Journal of Chronic Diseases, 30,* 302–322.

Dobson, K.S. (ed) (1988) *Handbook of Cognitive Behavioral Therapies* , Guilford Press, New York.

Eisenberg, M.G. (1982) 'Introduction' in M.G. Eisenberg, C. Griggins, and R.J. Duval (eds), *Disabled People as Second-Class Citizens,* pp. xii–xix. Springer, New York.

Eisenberg, M.G., Griggins, C. and Duval, R.J. (eds) (1982) *Disabled People as Second-Class Citizens,* Springer, New York.

Ellis, A. (1962) *Reason and Emotion in Psychotherapy,* Lyle Stuart, New York.

Ellis, A. (1963, May) 'The Treatment of Psychotic and Borderline Psychotics with Rational-emotive Psychotherapy', Paper presented at the *Symposium on Therapeutic Methods with Schizophrenics,* V.A. Hospital, Battle Creek, MI.

Ellis, A. (1975) *How to Live with a Neurotic at Home and at Work* (rev. ed.), Crown Publishers, New York.

Ellis, A. (1976) 'The Biological Basis of Human Irrationality', *Journal of Individual Psychology, 32,* 145–168.

Ellis, A. (1979) 'The Issue of Force and Energy in Behavioral Change', *Journal of Contemporary Psychotherapy, 10,* 83–97.

Ellis, A. (1980) 'Rational-emotive Therapy and Cognitive Behavior Therapy: Similarities and Differences', *Cognitive Therapy and Research, 4,* 325–340.

Ellis, A. and Bernard, M.E. (eds) (1985) *Clinical Applications of Rational-Emotive Therapy,* Plenum Press, New York.

Ellis, A. and Grieger, R. (eds) (1977) *Handbook of Rational-Emotive Therapy.* Springer, New York.

Ellis, A. and Harper, R.A. (1975) *A New Guide to Rational Living.* Prentice-Hall, Englewood Cliffs, NJ.

Ellis, A., McInerney, J.F., DiGiuseppe, R. and Yeager, R.J. (1988) *Rational-Emotive Therapy with Alcoholics and Substance Abusers,* Pergamon Press, New York.

Epstein, N., Schlesinger, S.E. and Dryden, W. (eds), (1988) *Cognitive-Behavioural Therapy with Families,* Brunner/Mazel, New York.

Evans, R.L., Halar, E.M. and Smith, K.M. (1985) 'Cognitive Therapy to Achieve Personal Goals: Results of Telephone Group Counseling with Disabled Adults', *Archives of Physical Medicine and Rehabilitation, 66,* 693–696.

Foreyt, J.P. and Rathjen, D.P. (eds) (1978) *Cognitive Behavior Therapy: Research and Applications,* Plenum Press, New York.

Freeman, A. (ed) (1983) *Cognitive Therapy With Couples and Groups,* Plenum Press, New York.

Freeman, A. and Greenwood, V. (eds) (1987) *Cognitive Therapy: Applications in Psychiatric and Medical Settings,* Human Sciences Press, New York.

Fuchs, C.Z. and Rehm, L.P. (1977) 'A Self-control Behavior Therapy Program for Depression', *Journal of Consulting and Clinical Psychology, 45,* 206–215.

Gandy, G.L. (1985) 'Frequent Misperceptions of Rational-emotive Therapy: An Overview for the Rehabilitation Counselor', *Journal of Applied Rehabilitation Counseling, 16(4),* 31–35.

Goldfried, M., Decenteceo, E. and Weinberg, L. (1974) 'Systematic Rational Restructuring as a Self-control Technique', *Behavior Therapy, 5,* 247–254.

Greenberg, L.S. and Safran, J.D. (1984) 'Integrating Effect and Cognition: A Perspective on Therapeutic Change', *Cognitive Therapy and Research*, 559–578.

Greenberg, L.S. and Safran, J.D. (1987) *Emotion and Psychotherapy*, Guilford Press, New York.

Ivey, A.E., Ivey, M.B. and Simek-Downing, L. (1987) *Counseling and Psychotherapy: Integrating Skills, Theory and Practice* (2nd ed), Prentice-Hall, Englewood Cliffs, NJ.

Jacques, M.E., Linkowski, D.C. and Sieka, F.L. (1970) 'Cultural Attitudes Toward Disability: Denmark, Greece, and the United States', *International Journal of Social Psychiatry*, 16, 54–62.

Kottke, F.J. (1982) 'Philosophic Considerations of Quality of Life for the Disabled', *Archives of Physical Medicine and Rehabilitation* 63, 60–62.

Larcombe, N.A. and Wilson, P.H. (1984) 'An Evaluation of Cognitive-behavior Therapy for Depression in Patients with Multiple Sclerosis', *British Journal of Psychiatry*, 145, 366–371.

Livneh, H. (1986) 'A Unified Approach to Existing Models of Adaptation to Disability: Part I - A Model of Adaptation', *Journal of Applied Rehabilitation Counseling*, 17, 5–16, 56.

Marinelli, R.P. and Dell Orto, A.E. (eds) (1977) *The Psychological and Social Impact of Physical Disability*, Springer Publishing Co., New York.

Mayer, J.D. and Eisenberg, M.G. (1982) 'Self-concept and the Spinal-cord-injured: An Investigation Using the Tennessee Self-concept Scale', *Journal of Consulting and Clinical Psychology*, 50, 604–605.

McDaniel, J.W. (1976) *Physical Disability and Human Behavior* (2nd ed), Pergamon Press, New York.

McLean, P.D. and Hakstian, A.R. (1979) 'Clinical Depression: Comparative Efficacy of Outpatient Treatments', *Journal of Consulting and Clinical Psychology*, 47, 818–836.

Meichenbaum, D. (1977) *Cognitive-Behaviour Modification: An Integrative Approach*, Plenum Press, New York.

Ostby, S.S. (1985) 'A National-emotive Perspective', *Journal of Applied Rehabilitation Counseling*, 16(3), 30–33.

Pearce, S. (1983) 'A Review of Cognitive-behavioural Methods for the Treatment of Chronic Pain', *Journal of Psychosomatic Research*, 27, 431–440.

Raimy, V. (1975) *Misunderstanding of the Self: Cognitive Psychotherapy and the Misconception Hypothesis*, Jossey-Bass, San Francisco.

Raimy, V. (1985) 'Misconceptions and the Cognitive Therapies', in
M.J. Mahoney and A. Freeman (eds), *Cognition and Psychotherapy*, pp. 203–222, Plenum Press, New York.

Roeher, G.A. (1961) 'Significance of Public Attitudes in the
Rehabilitation of the Disabled', *Rehabilitation Literature, 22,*
66–72.

Rush, A.J., Beck, A.T., Kovacs, M. and Hollon, S. D. (1977)
'Comparative Efficacy of Cognitive Therapy and
Pharmacotherapy in the Treatment of Depressed Outpatients',
Cognitive Therapy and Research, 1, 17–37.

Safran, J.D. and Greenberg, L.S. (1987) 'Affect and the Unconscious:
A Cognitive Perspective' in R. Stern (ed), *Theories of the
Unconscious.,* (pp. 191–212), Analytic Press, Hillsdale, NJ.

Schneider, C.R. and Anderson, W. (1980) 'Attitudes Toward the
Stigmatized: Some Insights from Recent Research',
Rehabilitation Counseling Bulletin, 23, 299–313.

Shaw, B.F. (1980) 'Predictors of Successful Outcome in Cognitive
Therapy: A Pilot Study', Paper Presented at the Meeting of the
World Congress on Behavior Therapy, Jerusalem.

Smith, D. (1982) 'Trends in Counseling and Psychotherapy',
American Psychologist, 37, 802–809.

Tarrier, N., Maguire, P. and Kincey, J. (1983) 'Locus of Control and
Cognitive Behavior Therapy with Mastectomy Patients: A Pilot
Study', *British Journal of Medical Psychology, 56,* 265–270.

Thurer, S. (1980) 'Disability and Monstrosity: A Look at Literary
Distortions of Handicapping Conditions', *Rehabilitation
Literature, 41,* 12–15.

Vargo, J.W. (1978) 'Some Psychological Effects of Physical Disability',
American Journal of Occupational Therapy, 32(1), 31–34.

Vargo, J.W. (1985) 'The Nature and Effects of Attitudes on
Adjustment to Physical Disability', *Alberta Psychology, 14(5),*
5–6.

Vargo, J.W. (1986) 'The Role of Headwork in Rehabilitation', *Spinal
Columns,* August, 28–29.

Vargo, J.W. (1989) 'In the House of my Friend: Dealing with
Disability', *International Journal for the Advancement of
Counseling, 12,* 281–287.

Vash, C.L. (1981) *The Psychology of Disability,* Springer Publishing
Company, New York.

Vertes, R. (1971) 'The Should: A Critical Analysis', *Rational Living,*
6(2), 22–25.

Weinberg, J.S. (1987) 'Group Cognitive Behaviour Therapy for Sexual Rehabilitation of Spinal Cord-injured Clients' in A. Freeman and V. Greenwood (eds),*Cognitive Therapy: Applications in Psychiatric and Medical Settings* , (pp. 213–227), Human Sciences Press, New York.

Weinberg, D.G. and Santana, N.H. (1978) 'Comic Books: Champions of the Disabled Stereotype', *Rehabilitation Literature, 39,* 327–331.

Wessler, R.L. and Ellis, A. (1980) 'Supervision in Rational-emotive Therapy' in A.K. Hess, (ed), *Psychotherapy Supervision: Theory, Research and Practice* , (pp. 181–191), Wiley, New York.

Westwood, M.J. and Vargo, J.W. (1985) 'Counselling the Double-minority Status Client' in R.J. Samuda and A.W. Wolfgang (eds), *Intercultural Counselling and Assessment: Global Perspectives* (pp. 303–313), C.J. Hogrefe, Toronto.

Westwood, M.J., Vargo, J.W. and Vargo, F.A. (1981) 'Methods for Promoting Attitude Change Toward and Among Physically Disabled persons', *Journal of Applied Rehabilitation Counseling, 12,* 220–225.

Wetstein-Kroft, S.B. and Vargo, J.W. (1984) 'Children's Attitudes Towards Disability, A Review and Analysis of the Literature', *International Journal for the Advancement of Counselling, 7(3),* 181–195.

Wickless, C. and Kirsch, I. (1988) 'Cognitive Correlates of Anger, Anxiety, and Sadness', *Cognitive Therapy and Research, 12,* 367–377.

Wilson, P.H., Goldin, J.C. and Charbonneau-Powis, M. (1983) 'Comparative Efficacy of Behavioral and Cognitive Treatments of Depression', *Cognitive Therapy and Research, 7* , 111–124.

Wright, B.A. (1983) *Physical Disability: A Psychosocial Approach* , (2nd ed), Harper and Row, New York.

Chapter Five

ADAPTATION AND COPING STRATEGIES IN COUNSELLING

Keith F. Kennett

INTRODUCTION

The purpose of this chapter is to examine adaptation by both counsellor and client in rehabilitation counselling. A definition of rehabilitation counselling is given within an eclectic paradigm, and integrative models are presented. Rehabilitation counselling includes verbal discussions, individual assessment, programme development and decisions demonstrated by client choice, action and behaviour. In this chapter, rehabilitation counselling focuses upon adaptation, in terms of competence, competence building and coping strategies.

DEFINITION AND ECLECTIC APPROACH TO REHABILITATION COUNSELLING

Rehabilitation counselling, a special type of applied psychology, refers to the broad range of helping strategies, including behavioural, educational and social approaches, that enable individuals to overcome obstacles through effective organization. Individuals are encouraged to optimize personal resources and adapt in acceptable ways through the acquisition of competencies which employ effective coping strategies.

Rehabilitation counsellors are directly involved in helping clients acquire the actual skills necessary to deal adequately with stressful external demands. Such counselling assists individuals to adapt and act intentionally, thus enabling them to function more effectively within society.

Rehabilitation counselling does not simply involve the application of a basic science called psychology.

> Rather it involves consideration of a set of complex interrelationships between psychological theory, application, historic context, social influence, and the individual behaviour of the provider/applier and the recipient of such provisions or application (Goldstein and Krasner, 1987, p. 1).

The challenge of rehabilitation counselling rests with techniques now available. The once simple allegiance to a strict theory has been surpassed by a preponderance of therapists identifying with some form of eclecticism (Brabeck and Welfel, 1985). Smith (1982) acknowledged the openness and flexibility afforded by an eclectic model, but warned that the rejection of a single-theory approach may result in the confusion or a hodgepodge of inconsistent concepts and techniques (p. 802). Ward (1983) stated:

> Without guidelines to structure counselling and to govern the appropriate selection and application of theoretical demand, strategies and techniques, the eclectic faces the dangers of operating haphazardly, inconsistently, and less effectively than is desirable (p. 23).

It is important to understand the structure of the situation (the person and the environment), and to grasp the structure of the discipline, so that the counsellor is able to perceive interrelations and encourage a strong foundation for understanding between consumer and counsellor in setting goals and agreeing on solutions. Rehabilitation counselling is reliant upon guidelines and integrating structures which aim to decrease discrete information or conflicting knowledge and to discourage practice within a narrow specialization.

INTEGRATIVE MODELS

Several commonalities (Goldfried, 1982; Highlen and Hill, 1984; Ivey, 1980; Mahoney, 1988) have provided the foundation for integrative, metatheoretical models (e.g., Beutler, 1983; Hart, 1983; Lazarus, 1976) as a way of structuring both the thinking and practices of eclectic counsellors. Within such metatheoretical models the structuring determines the method and direction of any application.

The eclectic approach selects relevant aspects of different theories, thus allowing for flexibility and adaptation, and provides the basis for a general theory. General theories (e.g., Howard, Nance and Myers, 1986; Ivey and Simek-Downing, 1980; Nelson-Jones, 1988) provide a framework into which many theories can be integrated. Such a framework permits the counsellor, over a period of time, to increase his or her options and to vary approaches to assessment and programming by integrating knowledge and experience, thus increasing the maturity or sophistication of any intervention (e.g., Thompson, 1986) and, ideally, its effectiveness. With an improved understanding of competing theories and actual experience in counselling (Tracey, Hays, Malone and Herman, 1988) the counsellor becomes more flexible and adaptive. According to Goldfried and Newman (1985) there are five themes of integration. The themes are:

1. Divergent modes of therapy have the potential to complement each other;
2. Focusing upon the overall interaction of cognition, emotion and behaviour of the client has many advantages over a single-dimensional approach;
3. Empirical findings and scrutiny must guide the selection of therapeutic procedures;
4. A common theoretical language is important; and
5. Commonalities need to be organized into a set of principles of therapeutic change.

Tracey *et al.*, (1988) observed that experienced counsellors compared with less experienced counsellors showed greater response variability as a function of what the client said, and it seems likely that there were increases in the range of strategies and time involved. These researchers identified two types of response learning amongst counsellors, namely, their proficiency in the use of certain responses (response acquisition) and their selection of appropriate responses (strategy acquisition).

Strategy acquisition involves the counsellor making changes in response flexibility and using a wide range of responses. The shift from learning how to respond, to knowing how to select an appropriate response for the benefit of the client involves a focus on strategy. Responses have to be selected depending on the individual and the circumstances, and a considerable degree of discretion may be required. Counsellors also need to develop discriminatory judgement and recognize that immediacy of response is only appropriate in some contexts. The counsellor has to learn to vary responses in harmony with the behaviour or disposition of the client. Strategy acquisition should be consistent with greater variability and flexibility by the counsellor (Tracey *et al.*, 1988).

Effective counselling involves the counsellor providing the appropriate type of environment for each client (Tracey *et al.*, 1988). This may include assisting with individualized programmes, monitoring and developing daily activities and supporting such implementation through close and constant communication. Effective counselling is also viewed as recognizing that meaning is defined from the viewpoint of the client rather than the counsellor; that is, there is a need to focus attention on the learner's behaviour (Weir, 1965) and on individual personal commitment. Strategy acquisition integrates such recognition. Although there is an initial strength in the selection of and preference for a single-theory approach, there is a long-term advantage in remaining open and flexible, adapting to change, accepting and integrating new knowledge, evaluating ideas and learning for their practical relevance (Brill, 1985). Within the structure of rehabilitation counselling there is a recognition that many solutions to the same problem(s) exist, that clients are unique individuals, and that alternative ways of helping may provide improved response capacity and increase the speed of acquiring a variety of new patterns of behaviour.

FOCUS ON INTEGRATIVE MODELS

The focus of rehabilitation counselling in this chapter is upon inter-relationships and integrative models. Many examples exist to support such an approach. Harrison (1979) observed that three theoretical orientations frequently used in treating children are parent training, family systems therapy, and individual psychodynamically oriented psychotherapy. Jackson and Beers (1988) noted that some reports on the treatment of children may support specific theoretical orientations such as parent training as a superior treatment modality, but their preference was to integrate the three major orientations listed by Harrison (1979). Their strategy focused upon parent-child and family interactions as integral components of both the diagnostic and counselling processes.

Jackson and Beers (1988) wrote of the integrated developmental, counselling and psychotherapy regimen explored. The core of their process was the provision of developmental and continuously focused feedback involving ongoing assessment of each family member's progress, and nature of the particular family as a functional system. Their findings suggest that early intervention (acquisition of coping strategies and competencies), using an integrative approach in the treatment of emotional and behavioural disorder may reduce any destructive impact on the child, the family, and subsequently school and interpersonal relationships.

Murgatroyd (1988) wrote extensively on reversal theory as an integrative framework for the practice of psychotherapy, and the practice of structural phenomenological psychotherapy in particular. Underlying his theory of practice and intervention, is the accepted use of different procedures. Counsellors may have a particular theoretical perspective but should be free to select and use a variety of particular techniques developed by other schools as appropriate (Dryden, 1987). This model, then, insists upon consistent theory but selects and uses a wide variety of techniques from other models, adapting them for different purposes consistent with the initial theoretical perspective of the counsellor.

Another promising integrative approach to helping, called choice therapy, presented by Nelson-Jones (1988) integrated a variety of existential-humanistic approaches. This respects the uniqueness of the individual while utilizing the specificity of behavioural and cognitive psychology. Choice therapy aims to achieve three interrelated goals, namely:

> to raise clients' awareness of the existential imperative that ultimately they are responsible for their choice in life, to help clients gain more self-esteem, and to facilitate and educate them in developing self-help skills of becoming better choosers in the areas they find problematic (p. 43).

Each integrative approach involves programmes and strategies that include the essential acquisition of competencies by the client. Social and cognitive skills must be acquired by the client in order to decide on goals, to become committed, to make effective behavioural selections, and thus act competently. The understanding of the meaning of adaptive counselling and the developmental process is essential in rehabilitation counselling.

ADAPTIVE COUNSELLING, THERAPY AND THE DEVELOPMENTAL PROCESS

There are numerous models that support inter-relatedness and integrative approaches but, of particular interest is one founded on principles of adaptive behaviour. Howard *et al.*, (1986) presented an important integrative approach called the Adaptive Counselling and Therapy (ACT) model, which is based on the task-relevant developmental maturity of the client. This approach focuses upon the developmental process. Clients are helped to grow from one level of maturity to a higher level of developmental maturity, with the counselling assisting the client's upward movement. Such developments are essential for the optimization of personal resources and the acquisition and building of competencies and increased personal adaptability.

> The developmentally advanced individual possesses a wide range of modes of responding that are both differentiated from each other and hierarchically organized (and) provides an increased flexibility as well as stability at higher levels. Multiple means become available for achievement of a particular goal and multiple goals can be served by a single means (Zigler and Glick, 1986).

The understanding of developmental processes is a prerequisite in helping clients (e.g., Cicchetti and Schneider-Rosen, 1983; Wode, 1983), and clarifying "the relationship between separate areas of development such as cognitive, social and linguistic developments" (Lewis, 1987). The possession of competencies by individuals is more or less developed, acquired, and integrated during successive periods of life (Masterpasqua, 1989). For example, Stern (1985) demonstrated that nonverbal interpersonal synchrony and trust in dyadic relatedness commenced in infancy and were later subsumed under more abstract forms of adaptation, while their relevance, in terms of adjustment, continued to apply.

Competence has been defined as those "personal characteristics (knowledge, skills and attitudes) which lead to adaptive payoffs in significant environments" (Sundberg, Snowden and Reynolds, 1978, p. 126) and as "learned attitudes and aptitudes, manifested as capacities for confronting, actively struggling with and mastering life problems through the use of cognitive and social skills" (Caplan, 1980, p. 671).

The identification and promotion of significant and adaptive competencies are the primary concern of counsellors in assisting clients to overcome problems and prevent other difficulties. Bloom (1979) reached a similar conclusion, stating: "Of all explanatory concepts that have been introduced to link problems to characteristics of the social system, the most compelling have been the concepts of competence and competence building" (p. 184).

Descriptions of competencies, typically acquired during different stages of the life span, are important (Scroufe and Rutter, 1984). These include, for example, flexible self-control during early childhood and an integrative life during old age. Such descriptions can serve as constituents of a self-organizing system. In addition, these descriptions can serve as diagnostic criteria in comparing the individual with others in terms of competence and competence deficits. Scroufe and Rutter (1984) focused understanding on the interplay between patterns of adaptation and maladaptation during developmental periods within the life cycle, and identified childhood symptoms that may be predictors of adult psychopathology. Similarly, Kohlberg, Ricks, and Snarey (1984), in refining this position, concluded that patterns of adaptational competencies in contrast to symptoms may be more accurate indicators or predictors of the emergence of maladjustment.

Such broad-based indicators of adaptational failure as inadequate peer relations, antisocial behaviour, and achievement problems during the school years do predict adult disorders with some power (Scroufe and Rutter, 1984). These indicators are of an integrative nature and include developmental socioemotional and cognitive aspects of the individual.

Counselling initially helps in the development of specific responses in social settings. Individuals gain competencies which develop and become integrated into response patterns during successive periods of life, with earlier acquired competencies maintaining their significance for adjustment. "Optimal development more accurately consists of the individual's active reorganization and integration of the various competencies acquired through the life span" (Masterpasqua, 1989).

The life span perspective of development, and the recognition that continuing psychological adjustment depends on competencies and the organization of component skills into viable systems (Masterpasqua, 1989), lead to a model in which competencies are placed within a constructivist-developmental framework. In mental health counselling, Mahoney (1988) noted that viability of self, rather than rational thought, was a central issue. The viability of the individual depends on self-help skills and personal and social responsibilities, which allow individuals to cope successfully with the demands of life. This is the ultimate goal of counselling. The ability to seek many changes in many situations involves a re-examination of the current problem and the acquisition of new or improved skills to resolve old and current issues.

An underlying function and a basic goal of all counselling is to increase the client's response capacity, that is, the ability to generate or create new behaviours and thoughts (Ivey and Simek-Downing, 1980), to generalize (Ward, 1989), and to become independent as a decision-maker, who has personal commitment. Existing and new coping strategies assist in reaching such effective adaptive behaviour.

The Adaptive Counselling and Therapy (ACT) model (Howard, *et al.*, 1986) provides the concept of match and move, in which accurate matching of the client's current needs is determined by the level of task-relevant developmental maturity, which optimizes the therapeutic progress by maximizing the client's movement towards higher maturity levels. In this model, counsellor styles are identified: telling, teaching, supporting and delegating. The ACT model underpins the major thrust in the process of normalization as the key issues in rehabilitation counselling, while maintaining a generic approach to all forms of counselling. Gabbard, Howard and Dunfee (1980) investigated counsellor adaptability, and their findings support the view that ACT theory is highly predictive of counselling outcome, and is related to counsellor constructs such as empathy, and talkativeness.

ADAPTIVE BEHAVIOUR IN TERMS OF PERSON-ENVIRONMENT FIT

Sundberg (1977) viewed behaviour as a function of both person and environment. Knowing what personal resources currently exist, how to develop further resources in terms of competencies and skills, and where and when these resources will be needed in terms of the demands of each specific environment are relevant and important. The specific resources of the individual must be constantly matched with the demands of the environment along with an understanding of those demands. It is the skill of helping the individual match personal resources with environmental demands which constitutes the process of rehabilitation counselling. The counsellor helps through verbal discussions that focus on understanding the demands encountered by the client. He or she also assists in the design and implementation of programmes of action based upon individual assessment and evaluation.

ASSESSMENT

Assessment is a process that describes an individual at a particular point in time and infers what an individual can do currently (Kennett, 1975). From such an assessment, predictions can be made regarding individual performance in the future, a profile can be made in terms of current strengths and deficits, along with objective monitoring of individual progress which can be compared against self, a group of similar individuals in counselling and against norms of age-related behaviours (Kennett, 1977a).

Assessment Instruments

A number of assessment instruments have been developed for use in rehabilitation counselling. In the field of developmental disabilities there are many examples (e.g. Gunzburg, 1968; Marlett, 1971; Nihira, Foster, Shellhaas and Leland, 1974). Gunzburg (1968) concluded that the content of rehabilitation programmes should be social education and set about reducing social inadequacy through assessment of individual attainment in the field of social knowledge and competence (The Progress Assessment Chart of Social Development) and subsequent programmes that fitted individual needs. Marlett (1971) developed the Adaptive Functioning Index, another practical measure of current behaviours that focuses upon independent functioning in the areas of social education, vocational skills and home living skills. The AAMD Adaptive Behaviour Scales (Nihira *et al.*, 1974) provide an assessment of social awareness and social competency. The process involves diagnosis and classification including possible interpretations of the relationship between various domains and sub-domains as observed and reported in similar and different environments (Kennett, 1985a).

Assessment measures provide information on current client behaviour to enable the counsellor to assist and advise on how best to match personal resources with environmental situations and opportunities. Such assessments have become an important requirement in the process of identification and placement. The adaptation scales serve to assist in knowing what behaviours to teach in order to facilitate the transition of clients into integrated, learning and living environments (Kennett, 1985b), and in decreasing bias often associated with other assessments dependent on school-type behaviours. They highlight opportunities for including parents, spouses and the client in effective educational planning (Bruininks, McGrew, and Maruyama, 1988).

Research involving individuals with autism has demonstrated the importance of counsellor knowledge of client and environment (Kennett and Kennett, 1982). Because of the complexities of behaviours displayed by the individual with autism (e.g., abnormal multi-dimensional behaviours including social contact, attention span, style and level of communication), the counsellor may, in the beginning, be at a loss. "For persons with autism, adaptive behaviour may be an area of significant need given the impairments of communication and social skills associated with the syndrome" (Loveland and Kelley, 1988).

Individualized programmes often involve multiple areas of assessment (Brown and Hughson, 1987; Close and Foss, 1988; Halpern, Nave, Close and Nelson, 1986; Kennett, 1981a; Kennett and Kennett, 1982; Parmenter, 1988; Whelan, Speake and Strickland, 1984) for counsellors working with individuals with autism. These include adaptive behaviour, evaluations of quality of treatment, medical reports and goals based on behavioural objectives. Halpern, Nave, Close and Nelson (1986) developed an integrated model of community adjustment and included four key dimensions of transition from school to adult life, namely, occupation, residential environment, social support and personal satisfaction. They developed a battery of tests which examine three variables in each of the four dimensions. Such multi-disciplinary and multi-dimensional approaches to the assessment process (Brown and Hughson, 1987; Mitchell, 1986) provide a basis for effective interpretation and meaningful prescription. The measurement techniques can assess the client's cognitive abilities, current level of coping with the social and natural demands of the general environment and the expectations of specific environments, such as the school, home or residence.

Profiles for individual development include knowing what personal resources currently exist, knowing how to develop further resources in terms of competencies and skills, and knowing when and where these resources would be needed in terms of specific environments (Kennett, 1981b). In other words, the counsellor must be knowledgeable about the system in which the individual functions or might function. Different environments may define competence in various ways, thus requiring a classification system that would include identification of the adaptation needs in real-life situations, or ecologically valid settings (Lowitzer, Utley and Baumeister, 1987).

Provision of the appropriate type of environment implies knowing what is needed and what actually exists. For example, the appropriate type of home environment involves an assessment of the family members and the degree to which the home environment reflects the norms of societal behaviour. It must take into account the uniqueness of the family unit (Kennett, 1979). Rehabilitation counsellors need to be accepted by the family in order to obtain a comprehensive knowledge of the client's home. A quick evaluation of counsellor acceptance is indicated by an invitation to have a cup of coffee or tea, not in the front living room, but in the kitchen!

Assisting families necessitates individual assessment of each member in the family, and the interaction between them in order to know and understand the family constellation as a uniquely functioning unit. For example, in a particular home, the common eating practice may involve eating food with fingers, walking about while eating and drinking soup straight from the bowl. A different set of behaviours may be used by family members using knife, fork and soup spoon while seated at a table, in a different environmental setting outside of the home, such as a restaurant.

Individuals from cultural-familial restricted families must frequently acquire two sets of coping behaviours, one for the home and another for acceptance in the community. Similarly, movement from one culture to another involves different ways of doing things, including simple tasks like having a bath (Kennett, 1981c).

The family is a system that functions as part of a much wider system (Bronfenbrenner, 1979), managing resources and individual member differences, and accomplishing tasks both unique to the family unit and common to all families. The family is a system of interacting individuals each with its own strengths and weaknesses, collectively and individually (Gomersall, 1986). Knowing the strengths of a family may be crucial in bringing about meaningful change and further coping strategies. Knowing the family may also result in recognition that many cope with and adapt to the stresses encountered.

Furthermore, the examination of the family as a unit should recognize the family as consumers of services, and include a careful analysis of its component relationships to prevent the glossing over of critical family characteristics (Cole and Jordan, 1989). For example, the present author in his counselling practice devised a programme for a twelve year old female where behaviour was unexpected as she refused to acquire telephone skills and became quite violent when forced to pick up the telephone. Investigation of the home environment revealed that only father was permitted to pick up the telephone, as the telephone had only recently been connected. The reason for unacceptable behaviour by the twelve year old was suddenly observed as understandable within the home environment.

Adaptation refers to modification and adjustment to environments in order to survive, control and benefit from the environment. Olson, Russell and Sprenkle (1983) defined adaptability, in reference to the family, as the family's ability to change its rules, roles and power structure in response to stress. Degrees of adaptability are presented by Cole and Jordan (1989) in terms of low adaptability (or rigidity) and high adaptability (or chaos); this approach reflects high conformity on the one hand and high non-conformity on the other. Just as the authors demonstrate that "different components of the family may be more cohesive and adaptable than others", so adaptability may occur in both high conforming and high non-conforming ways, varying from situation to situation. Adaptation reflects the degree of successful modification and is judged on effective adjustment outcomes.

Much of what an individual learns is the product of observing the behaviour of others, especially those of the immediate family (Kennett, 1977b). The Family Behaviour Profile (Kennett, 1978), an assessment of the behavioural tendencies of all members of the family, provides information relating to the on-going daily experiences of the family. Counsellors, with such information, are better positioned to approach issues from both an individual and family system viewpoint.

Understanding the family constellation is essential in identifying strengths and weaknesses, in advising on learning programmes, and devising improved modelling techniques. Provision can be made to allow for the individuality of the family system, where family members evolve their own style of coping strategies using their own resources, thus adapting to their own family environment. Within defined and acceptable behavioural ranges, family deviations (adaptability) from expected modes of social conduct can be condoned, with the counsellor knowing, understanding, and recognizing that it is all right to be different (Kennett, 1979). Furthermore, such differences may vary with family members, where not all components of the family, especially in dysfunctional families, are equally cohesive or adaptable (Cole and Jordan, 1989).

Rehabilitation counselling, on the one hand, continues to

address the developmentally significant areas of competence deficits and, on the other hand, promotes those cognitive, behavioural and socioemotional characteristics which reduce the vulnerability of an individual in dealing with subsequent problems (Bond, 1984). In the process of reducing vulnerability the counsellor is also helping the client reduce or manage stress. The client may need to re-arrange events to reduce real or perceived adversity, thus making coping behaviours more effective. Coping and the classification of coping are important factors in the process of stress management and adaptive behaviour.

DEFINITION OF COPING

Coping, usually associated with stress, has been defined by Levine (1983) as an overly inclusive aggregate of behavioural and somatic response processes. Coping, according to Pearlin and Schooler (1982) are the things people do to avoid being harmed by life strains. A fundamental assumption is made that people are actively responsive to forces that impinge upon them. For example, Affleck, Tennen and Rowe (1988) examined risk and prevention appraisals reported by mothers after the birth of high-risk infants. These researchers drew attention to the importance of examining the psychological dimensions of risk including the provision of prevention appraisals in order to counsel parents more effectively about their future childbearing.

CLASSIFICATION OF COPING

According to Lazarus and Launier (1978) coping can be classified into the following four modes:

1. Information Seeking:
    an attempt to reappraise the situation or challenge upon which some form of action or response may depend;

2. Direct Action:
   a way of changing self or environment and thus meeting the challenge;

3. Inhibition of Action:
   a way of resisting action as being inappropriate;

4. Cognitive Coping:
   a strategy involving the manipulation of a person's attention, or re-arranging the way events are apprehended and thus bringing about a reduction of the perceived challenge.

Coping responses within stressful situations vary on two important information-seeking dimensions, namely, "monitoring (which) involves the extent to which individuals are alert for and sensitized to information about threat" and "blunting (which) involves the extent to which individuals distract themselves from and psychologically blunt threatening cues" (Miller, Leinbach and Brody, 1989).

The classification of coping for clients has many similarities to the steps in the counselling or problem-solving process. The counselling process usually involves "building the relationship and identifying client concerns, establishing realistic counselling goals, designing effective procedures (such as monitoring and blunting), and terminating the counselling process" (Hutchins and Meo, 1987).

Dixon and Glover (1984) in their problem-solving model prefer not to provide discrete stages in the counselling process but rather to indicate benchmarks for analyzing and understanding successful counselling. These authors examine the processes of problem definition, goal selection (information seeking), strategy selection, implementation of strategy (direct or inhibited action), and evaluation (cognitive coping). Similarly, Georgiades and Phillimore (1975), in an examination of the counselling process, have previously highlighted the need to define the problem, set goals, gain consensus from key personnel (notwithstanding that such consensus can be overridden by the choice of the client), identify a group to implement change and evaluate progress.

COPING STRATEGIES

An examination of the types of coping strategies involves an examination of the environment, interaction with others, the social support system, the personal characteristics of the consumer as well as his or her skills in cognitive and social acquisition. Rehabilitation programmes need to be evaluated in terms of a person's improved quality of life including how clients perceive this improvement (Brown, Bayer and MacFarlane, 1989).

Some systematic research has focused on family stress and coping as children approach adulthood (Suelzle and Keenan, 1981; Wikler, 1986). Like previous researchers, Donovan (1988) acknowledged that families change over time and that an understanding of the growth and change that occurs throughout the lifecycle of a family is important.

Family reaction to stress is highly variable, ranging from effective adaptation to maladaptation. Recent models of family adaptation to stress (e.g. Crnic, Friedrich and Greenberg, 1983; Hill, 1949; McCubbin and Patterson, 1983) explain such variability. Adaptation models centre upon the role of coping behaviour in mediating stress. Stress can result in distress, and stress can influence the acquisition of more resources or better utilization of existing resources to make family members sufficiently equipped to handle the situations. Boss (1988) illustrated that there can be positive effects of crisis (in contrast to stress) as a means of facilitating family change, under very skilled counselling. Donovan (1988), using this adaptation approach, reported on mother's perceptions of family stress and ways of coping with adolescents who were autistic or had other developmental disabilities, and concluded that child-related stress was higher, as perceived by mothers of autistic adolescents, than other mothers. However, maternal coping styles, despite heavy reliance on community resources and professional help for coping, were consistent across groups. Community services and programmes are essential in successful maternal adaptation to a child with developmental disabilities. Mothers coped more successfully when such services were perceived as helpful. Under such circumstances professionals, such as counsellors, contributed to healthy family adaptation by carefully monitoring how parents perceived their programmes and by responding to the needs families identify (Donovan, 1988). Another study by Byrne and Cunningham (1988) found that providing financial and/or practical services was insufficient. Alleviation of stress and the enhancement of life involved interventions that focused upon relationships among family members, supported family cohesiveness and encouraged all family members to participate in family activities and decisions.

In Donovan's 1988 study, when the demands of parenting exceeded the resources of the family, mothers coped by actively seeking assistance outside of the family system. For those mothers whose life events and stresses were associated with low social economic status rather than marital relationships, reliance was directed more on service resources and programmes. Such mothers used [strategies] less frequently and found less helpful those strategies that focused upon an optimistic definition of the situation, the mobilization of family resources, and insisted upon the maintenance and improvement of their own psychological well-being.

Environments can be designed, for example in prisons where offenders are largely poor copers, to promote self-review and inspire self-reform. Again, programmes designed by counsellors must explicitly teach coping skills, decision-making skills and organizational strategies including short-term solutions to problems as well as long-term planning. Such programmes include training in ways to analyze problem situations, with evaluation and projection of the likely consequences of proposed actions. Consumers need to acquire techniques such as cognitive restructuring, problem-solving, covert responding, and anticipatory skills. Attention must be given to the conditions for promoting transfer of new skills to and within the natural environment (Zamble and Porporino, 1988).

Similarly, Kennett (1976) demonstrated the importance of promoting the transfer of new skills acquired by persons, predominantly with cultural-familial disabilities, participating in a Work Adjustment Training Programme. Those clients who had experienced long-term unemployment not only gained new work skills, but also new social skills and competencies. Work habits and skills were enhanced and consolidated as a result of the heavy emphasis on counselling that focused upon individual needs for personal, social and work competence, and the provision of realistic goals with minimization of conflict in goal selection.

The Work Adjustment Assessment Profile (Kennett, 1976) makes it possible to examine adaptive behaviours in terms of coping strategies and competencies in the areas of general work skills, work habits and routine, personal qualities and strengths, learning and social behaviour. The transfer of these behaviours was examined and found to be necessary and relevant in terms of application to work experience, on the job training and real employment applications.

Ward (1989) cautioned the counsellor in regard to the exacting task of skill transfer, especially in the areas of generalization and vertical transfer, while maintaining a conviction that some training programmes improve status and performance, and bring clients with developmental disabilities closer to normal functioning levels. In reviewing programmes that reported on the acquisition and use of generalizable skills and strategies in persons having developmental disabilities, Ward (1989) concluded that current instructional technology has achieved somewhat modest results while acknowledging the benefits to clients of challenging training environments.

Research by Kennedy, Fisher and Pearson (1988) demonstrated the importance of interaction with others. They used a behavioural mapping procedure to examine a pattern of interaction and location of patient and staff in a rehabilitation unit for traumatically spinal cord injured people. Their findings support the view that interaction with others (including group interaction) and relation between feedback and behaviour are very important in rehabilitation counselling.

Coping with daily routine means encounters with others, and places the individual in regular situations of cooperation and support on the one hand, and conflict and isolation on the other hand. Recent research (Rynders, Schleien and Mustonen, 1990) provided a learning environment to assist individuals with severe disabilities cope better by the acquisition of cooperative learning strategies. The study demonstrated that social interaction, including positive reinforcement and co-operative learning strategies can be promoted by integrating children with severe disabilities in an intensified outdoor education programme, in the form of organized camping. The coping strategies of both individuals without disabilities and those with severe disabilities were modified and adjusted such that there was increased social interaction, positive perceptions of friendship by campers without disabilities, and positive staff member ratings concerning integrated camping experiences. Skills, especially social coping skills, are best achieved with the participation of significant others, such as peers. Similar findings were reported by Kennett and Buchanan (1973) where school activities focused upon meaningful skill acquisition through inter-disciplinary approaches, positive peer support and participation.

Kennett and Buchanan (1973) demonstrated the importance of physical education in the lower elementary grades as an essential activity appropriate to the effective development of each student. The learning environment allowed students of widely varying skills and abilities to participate and enjoy the processes of education. Rehabilitation counselling was in action. For example, one student aged seven with cerebral palsy (limited muscular and body coordination but mobile) participated like all other students in the physical education programme. His high level of motivation and determination to do things with his peer group led to improved muscular coordination as well as peer acceptance and high positive self-esteem. Similarly, another student with learning difficulties who showed serious withdrawal symptoms and rarely participated in regular class activities, developed significant behavioural changes because of new competencies gained with peer support. At the end of the twenty week programme she was challenging other students in competitive and social activities and had developed substantial leadership skills.

Counselling may involve indirect approaches in social settings where peer support and peer participation are essential for the learning of personal and social competencies in coping.

Social support is an important coping resource and is essential for individuals experiencing stressful life changes (Cohen and Wills, 1985). Mallinckrodt (1989) contended that social support is multidimensional and functions in a stressor-specific manner. "Different types of support provide different coping resources, and because stressors vary in adaptational demands, a given type of support will be effective only when the coping resources it provides are matched to the demands of the stressor".

"Coping cannot be understood as a single, static response to a single demand but can only be properly understood in a transactional sense as a changing constellation of processes" (Wrubel, Benner and Lazarus, 1981, p. 68). The counsellor guides clients towards effective coping mechanisms and the acquisition of strategies to solve problems.

To some extent, coping is a temporally and situationally specific process (Folkman and Lazarus, 1980; Stone and Neale, 1984). Peterson (1989) noted that an individual may not respond to related situations in a similar fashion. He demonstrated, for example, that an individual who appears to cope with the news that surgery is necessary may cope differently when entering the operating room or when in the post-operative situation.

Measurement of coping in childhood where there are developmental disabilities has a further level of complexity, resulting from substantial shifts in development. The coping process being assessed may occur at a time of potential and actual rapid change in individual client perceptions and abilities. Coping may be demonstrated in terms of individual approaches to environmental demands and also in terms of culturally determined response patterns. Those clients who differ from the mainstream or dominant culture (or race) may approach demands in different ways (Kennett, 1981c). A very delicate balance exists between individual and cultural aspects of response patterns and demonstrate different ways of coping or not coping.

Smith (1977) on the one hand reminds counsellors that "In an effort to sensitize others to the situations of members of a particular racial group, we sometimes ignore individual differences – defeating the very goals we set out to accomplish ". On the other hand, cultural differences involve an understanding and respect for alternate value systems. Wrenn (1976) listed respect for authority figures, the value of adults' past experiences, the role of women in culture, attitudes to sexuality, attitudes towards work and leisure, emphasis on economic and personal security, and attitudes towards occupational choice as examples where major differences may occur. Sue and Sue (1977) summarized these differences in terms of language barriers, class-bound values, and cultural-bound barriers. Sue (1978) provided guidelines to encourage culturally effective counselling. Counsellors should realize that others are different. They should avoid being culturally encapsulated, and draw on techniques and methods of counselling appropriate to the culture and lifestyle of the client. Even age and gender appropriateness and adaptive skills are acquired socially (Loveland and Kelley, 1988).

Coping strategies demonstrated by clients depend not only on environments, cultural differences in social group support and counsellor skill and experience, but on major personal qualities, such as motivation, determination and persistence of the client as well. Successful personal adaptation depends on at least three components, namely the clients' capabilities and skills to deal with the social and environmental demands (coping capabilities), motivation to meet these demands and their capabilities to maintain a state of psychological equilibrium so their energies and skills can be directed to external, in contrast to internal, needs (Mechanic, 1974).

Successful coping strategies are also influenced by other variables – personal style of the client; the degree to which the client wants to change and improve behaviour; the individual's desire for group and peer acceptance; how supportive environments which add personal client value are selected; and the extent to which the client demonstrates psychological equilibrium in dealing with internal and external needs, and shares responsibility.

Coping strategies permit the client to acquire a range of competencies essential for the ongoing acquisition of adaptive behaviours. Research in adaptive behaviour has paid special attention to the acquisition of social competencies as a priority in education and counselling. By embedding individual problems in a socio-psychological matrix the competence paradigm can "serve to rally psychologists around the goal of advocating for the personal empowerment of all individuals [providing] a clearer health-based, psychological alternative to the traditional disease-based medical model" (Masterpasqua, 1989).

The opportunity to maximize competencies and coping skills to deal with stress increases lifestyle efficiencies. Rehabilitation counselling identifies abilities that ensure a client's successful adaptation to the demands of the social and physical environment. Adaptation and coping strategies rely upon the competencies of both the counsellor and client and are demonstrated through theoretical constructs and in personal strategies that acknowledge that there are many ways of dealing with problems in life. Adaptation and coping strategies require the consideration and implementation of new ideas and approaches, and are involved in ongoing learning, and the development of sufficient knowledge to evaluate ideas and actions. Rehabilitation counselling helps overcome problems and prevents others; such counselling "is proactive in that it seeks to build adaptive strengths, coping resources, and health in people and primary prevention assumes that equipping people with personal and environmental resources for coping is the best of all ways" (President's Commission on Mental Health Report, 1978, p. 1833).

RECOMMENDATIONS

Rehabilitation counselling is defined within an eclectic paradigm supported by integrative models. Successful counselling depends on the unique qualities and personal style of each counsellor. Similarly, the client's commitment, motivation and independence to make decisions influences the level of success. Counselling relies on the different approaches taken to find ways of solving problems and dealing with stress. Finally, key items relating to the counsellor's role are summarized in point form:

1. Adaptive behaviour on the part of both the counsellor and

client are pre-requisites for success;

2. Structuring should be carefully examined, as this greatly determines the method and direction of influence and application;

3. The counsellor's role is to help the client optimize personal resources, and adapt and acquire competencies that are utilized in coping strategies;

4. To achieve these goals, the counsellor is compelled to be involved actively in individual assessment sessions, in programme development, decision-making and evaluation;

5. Counsellors should be aware of the client's response acquisition, the degree of proficiency in using certain responses, and the development of strategy acquisition.

6. Many solutions to the same problem(s) exist and each client may decide to take one of many different routes to problem solving. Counsellors are important in assisting clients to find these routes;

7. Coping strategies should be evaluated in terms of how the individual has used such strategies to improve quality of life as an outcome measure of the effectiveness of rehabilitation programmes;

8. The constant challenge of counselling is to increase the client's response capacity, that is, the ability to generate or create new behaviours and thoughts.

REFERENCES

Affleck, G., Tennen, H. and Rowe, J. (1988) 'Adaptational Features of Mothers' Risk and Prevention Appraisals after the Birth of High-Risk Infants', *American Journal of Mental Retardation*, 92, 360-368.

Beutler, L.E. (1983) *Eclectic Psychotherapy; a Systematic Approach.* Permagon, New York.

Bloom, B.L. (1979) 'Prevention of Mental Health Disorders: Recent Advances in Theory and Practice', *Community Mental Health Journal*, 15, 179-191.

Bond, L.A. (1984) 'From Prevention to Promotion: Optimizing Infant Development' in J. M. Joffee, G.W. Albee and L.D. Kelly (eds), *Readings in Primary Prevention of Psychopathology*, University Press of New England, Hanover, NH.

Boss, P.G. (1988) *Family Stress Management*, Newbury Park, Sage.

Brabeck, M.M., and Welfel, E.R. (1985) 'Counseling Theory: Understanding the Trend Towards Eclecticism from a Developmental Perspective', *Journal of Counseling and Development*, 63, 343-348.

Brill, N.I. (1985) *Working with People: The Helping Process*, Longman, New York.

Brofenbrenner, U. (1979) *The Ecology of Human Development*, Harvard University Press, Cambridge, Massachussetts.

Brown, R.I., Bayer, M. and MacFarlane, C. (1989) *Rehabilitation Programmes: Performance and Quality of Life of Adults with Developmental Handicaps*, Lugus Productions Ltd., Toronto, Ontario.

Brown, R.I. and Hughson, E.A. (1987) *Behavioral and Social Rehabilitation and Training*, John Wiley, New York.

Bruininks, R., McGrew, K. and Maruyama, G. (1988) 'Structure of Adaptive Behavior in Samples with and without Mental Retardation', *American Jourrnal of Mental Retardation*, 93, 265-272.

Byrne E.A. and Cunningham, C.C. (1988) 'Lifestyle and Satisfaction in Families of Children with Down's Syndrome', in R.I. Brown (ed), *Quality of Life and Rehabilitation.* Croom Helm, London.

Caplan, G. (1980) 'An Approach to Preventive Intervention in Developmental Psychology', *Canadian Journal of Psychology*, 25, 671-682.

Cicchetti, D. and Schneider-Rosen, K. (1983) 'Theoretical and Empirical Considerations in the Investigation of the Relationship between Affect and Cognition in Atypical Populations of Infants', in C. Izard, J. Kagan and R. Zajonc (eds), *Emotions, Cognition and Behaviour*, Cambridge University Press, New York.

Close, D.W. and Foss, G. (1988) 'Approaches to Training the Social Skills Needed for Quality of Life', in R.I. Brown (ed), *Quality of Life and Rehabilitation,* Croom Helm, London.

Cohen, S. and Wills, T.A. (1985) 'Stress, Social Support, and the Buffering Hypothesis', *Psychological Bulletin, 98,* 310-357.

Cole, D. A. and Jordan, A.E. (1989) 'Assessment of Cohesion and Adaptability in Component Family Dyads: A Question of Convergent and Discriminant Validity', *Journal of Counseling Psychology, 36,* 456-463.

Crnic, K.A., Friedrich, W.N. and Greenberg, M.T. (1983) 'Adaptation of Families with Mentally Retarded Children: A Model of Stress, Coping and Family Ecology', *American Journal of Mental Deficiency, 88,* 125-138.

Donovan, A.M. (1988) 'Family Stress and Ways of Coping with Adolescents who have Handicaps: Maternal Perceptions', *American Journal of Mental Retardation, 92,* 502-509.

Dixon, D.N. and Glover, J.A. (1984) *Counseling: A Problem-Solving Approach,* John Wiley, New York.

Dryden, W. (1987) 'Theoretically Consistent Eclecticism - Humanizing a Computer Addict', in J. Norcross (ed), *Casebook of Eclectic Psychotherapy,* Brunner /Mazel, New York.

Folkman, S. and Lazarus, R. S. (1980) 'An Analysis of Coping in a Middle Aged Community Sample', *Journal of Health and Social Behavior, 21,* 219 - 239.

Gabbard, C.E., Howard, G.S. and Dunfee, E.J. (1980) 'Reliability, Sensitivity to Measuring Change, and Construct Validity of a Measure of Counselor Adaptability', *Journal of Counseling Psychology, 33,* 377-386.

Georgiades, N.J. and Phillimore, L. (1975) 'The Myth of Hero-innovator and Alternative Strategies for Organizational Change', in C.C. Kierna and F.D. Woodford (eds), *Behaviour Modification with the Severely Retarded,* Associated Scientific Publishers, Amsterdam.

Goldfried, M.P. (1982) 'Towards the Delineation of Therapeutic Change Principles', *American Psychologist, 35,* 991-999.

Goldfried, M.P., and Newman, C. (1985) 'Psychotherapy Integration - A Historic Perspective', in J. Norcross (ed), *Handbook of Eclectic Psychotherapy,* Brunner/Mazel, New York.

Goldstein, A.P. and Krasner, L. (1987) *Modern Applied Psychology,* Praeger, New York.

Gomersall, J.D. (1986) 'The Art of Therapy in a Family Where There is a Handicapped Member', in J.M. Berg (ed), *Science and Service in Mental Retardation*, Methuen, London.

Gunzburg, H.C. (1968) *Social Competence and Mental Handicap*, Bailliere, Tindall and Cassell, London.

Halpern, A.S., Nave, G., Close, D.W. and Nelson, D. (1986) 'An Empirical Analysis of the Dimensions of Community Adjustment for Adults with Mental Retardation in Semi-independent Living Programmes', *Australia and New Zealand Journal of Developmental Disabilities*, 12, 147-157.

Harrison, S.I. (1979) 'Child Psychiatric Treatment: Status and Prospectus', in J.D. Noshpitz (ed), *Basic Handbook of Child Psychiatry*, Basic Books, New York.

Hart, J.T. (1983) *Modern Eclectic Counseling: a Functional Orientation*, Plenum Press, New York.

Highlen, P.S. and Hill, C.E. (1984) 'Factors Affecting Client Change in Individual Counseling: Current Status and Theoretical Speculations', in S.D. Brown and R.W. Lent, *Handbook of Counseling Psychology*, Wiley, New York.

Hill, R. (1949) *Families under Stress*, Harper and Row, New York.

Howard, G.S., Nance, D.W. and Myers, P. (1986) 'Adaptive Counseling and Therapy: an Integrative Eclectic Approach', *The Counseling Psychologists*, 14, 363-442.

Hutchins, D.E. and Meo, K.K. (1987) 'Counselling Theories and Techniques' in C.W. Humes (ed) *Contemporary Counseling: Services, Applications, Issues*, Accelerated Development, Muncie, Indiana.

Ivey, A.E. (1980) 'Counseling 2000: Time to Take Charge', *The Counseling Psychologist*, 8, 12-16.

Ivey, A.E. and Simek-Downing, L. (1980) *Counseling and Psychotherapy: Skills, Theories, and Practice*, Prentice-Hall, Englewood Cliffs, NJ.

Jackson, R.L. and Beers, P.A. (1988) 'Focused Videotape Feedback Psychotherapy: An Integrated Treatment for Emotionally and Behaviorally Disturbed Children', *Counseling Psychology Quarterly*, 1, 11-23.

Kennedy, P., Fisher, K. and Pearson, E. (1988) 'Ecological Evaluation of a Rehabilitative Environment for Spinal Cord Injured People: Behavioural Mapping and Feedback', *British Journal of Clinical Psychology*, 27, 239-246.

Kennett, K.F. and Buchanan, C.R. (1973) 'Learning Experiences Through Physical Education', Paper presented at the *Annual Conference of the Atlantic Provinces Health, Physical Education and Recreation Association*, University of Moncton, Moncton, NB.

Kennett, K.F. (1975) 'The Adaptive Behavior Scales: New Uses and the Family Behavior Profile', Paper presented at the *83rd Annual Convention of the American Psychological Association*, Chicago.

Kennett, K.F. (1976) *The Work Adjustment Assessment Profile*, St. Francis Xavier University, Sydney, N.S.

Kennett, K.F. (1977a) 'The Family Behavior Profile: an Initial Report', *Mental Retardation, 15*, 36-40.

Kennett, K.F. (1977b) 'Adaptive Behavior and its Assessment,' in P. Mittler (ed), *Research to Practice in Mental Retardation* (Vol. II), University Park Press, Baltimore.

Kennett, K.F. (1978) *The Family Behavior Profile: Test and Manual* (Revision), Nepean College of Advanced Education, Sydney.

Kennett, K.F. (1979) 'The Family Behavior Profile: an Initial Report', in L. Baruth and M. Burgraf, *Readings in Counseling Parents of Exceptional Children*, Special Learning Corporation, Guilford, New York.

Kennett, K.F. (1981a) 'Matching the Resources of Developmentally Disabled with the Demands of Specific Environments', Paper presented at the *Sixteenth Annual Conference of the Australian Psychological Society*, Sydney.

Kennett, K.F. (1981b) 'Research into Adaptive Behaviour of Children with Developmental Handicaps', Paper presented at the *National Seminar on Research to Practice in the Habilitation of the Developmentally Handicapped*, Brisbane.

Kennett, K.F. (1981c) 'Assessing Adaptive Behaviors in the Developmentally Disabled: Cross-Cultural Implications', Paper presented at the *Joint International Council of Psychologists and International Association for Cross-Cultural Psychology Asian Conference*, National Taiwan University: Taiwan.

Kennett, K.F. and Kennett, B.E. (1982) 'Autism: Profiles for Individual Development at Home and School', Paper presented at the *6th Congress of the International Association for the Scientific Study of Mental Deficiency*, Toronto, Canada.

Kennett, K.F. (1985a) 'Assessing Adaptive Behaviour and Social Competence in the Family and Society', Paper presented at the *7th World Congress of the International Association for the Scientific Study of Mental Deficiency*, New Delhi.

Kennett, K.F. (1985b) 'Adult Independence, Residential and Employment Facilities for Autistic Adults', Paper presented at the *7th World Congress of the International Association for the Scientific Study of Mental Deficiency*, New Delhi.

Kohlberg, L., Ricks, D. and Snarey, J. (1984) 'Childhood Development as a Predictor of Adaptation in Adulthood', *Genetic Psychology Monograph, 110*, 91-172.

Lazarus, A.A. (1976) *Multimodal Behavior Therapy.*, Springer, New York.

Lazarus, R.S. and Launier, R. (1978) 'Stress-related Transactions Between Person and Environment', in L.A. Pervin and M. Lewis (eds), *Perspectives in Interactional Psychology*, Plenum, New York.

Levine, S. (1983) 'A Psychobiological Approach to the Ontogeny of Coping, in N. Garmezy and M. Rutter (eds), *Stress, Coping and Development in Children*, McGraw-Hill, New York.

Lewis, V. (1987) *Development and Handicap*, Basil Blackwell, Oxford.

Loveland, K.A. and Kelley, M.L. (1988) 'Development of Adaptive Behavior in Adolescents and Young Adults with Autism and Down Syndrome', *American Journal of Mental Retardation, 93*, 84-92.

Lowitzer, A.C., Utley, C.A. and Baumeister, A.A. (1987) AAMD's 1983 'Classification in Mental Retardation as Utilized by State Mental Retardation/Developmental Disabilities Agencies', *Mental Retardation, 25*, 287-291.

Mahoney, M.J. (1988) 'The Cognitive Sciences anɔ Psychotherapy; Patterns in a Developing Relationship,' in K.S. Dobson (ed), *Handbook of Cognitive-Behavioral Therapies*, Guilford, New York.

Mallinckrodt, B. (1989) 'Social Support and the Effectiveness of Group Therapy', *Journal of Counseling Psychology, 36*, 170-175.

Marlett, N.J. (1971; revised 1976) *Adaptive Functioning Index*, Vocational and Rehabilitation Research Institute, Calgary.

Masterpasqua, F. (1989) 'A Competence Paradigm for Psychological Practice', *American Psychologist, 44*, 1366-1371.

McCubbin, H.L. and Patterson, J.M. (1983) 'The Family Stress Process: The Double ABCX model of Adjustment and Adaptation', in H.I. McCubbin, M.S.B. Sussman and A. J. Patterson (eds), *Social Stress and the Family: Advances and Developments in Family Stress Theory and Research*, Haworth, New York.

Mechanic, D. (1974) 'Social Structure and Personal Adaptation: Some Neglected Dimensions', in G.V. Coelho, D.A. Hamburg and J. E. Adams (eds), *Coping and Adaptation*, Basic Books, New York.

Miller, S.M., Leinbach, A. and Brody, D.S. (1989) 'Coping Style in Hypertensive Patients: Nature and Consequences', *Journal of Consulting and Clinical Psychology, 57*, 333-337.

Mitchell, D.R. (1986) 'A Developmental Systems Approach to Planning and Evaluating Services for Persons with Handicaps' in R.I. Brown (ed), *Management and Administration of Rehabilitation Programmes*, Croom Helm, London.

Murgatroyd, S. (1988) 'Reversal Theory and Psychotherapy', *Counseling Psychology Quarterly, 1*, 57-74.

Nelson-Jones, R. (1988) *Practical Counselling and Helping Skills* (2nd ed), Holt, Rinehart and Winston, Sydney.

Nihira, K., Foster, R., Shellhaas, M. and Leland, H. (1974) *Adaptive Behavior Scales Manual* (rev. ed.), American Association on Mental Deficiency, Washington, D.C.

Olson, D.H., Russell, C. and Sprenkle, D. (1983) 'Circumplex Model of Marital and Family Systems: VI. Theoretical Update', *Family Process, 22*, 69-83.

Parmenter, T.R. (1988) 'An Analysis of the Dimensions of Quality of Life for People with Physical Disabilities', in R. I. Brown, (ed), *Quality of Life for Handicapped People*, Croom Helm, London.

Pearlin, L.I. and Schooler, C. (1982) 'The Structure of Coping', in H.I. McCubbin, A.E. Cauble and J.M. Patterson (eds), *Family stress, Coping and Social Support*, Thomas, Springfield, Il.,

Peterson, L. (1989) 'Coping by Children Undergoing Stressful Medical Procedures: Some Conceptual, Methodological and Therapeutic Issues', *Journal of Counselling and Clinical Psychology, 57*, 380-387.

President's Commission on Mental Health (1978) Report of the Task Panel on Prevention, U.S. Government Printing Office, Washington.

Rynders, J.E., Schleien, S.J. and Mustonen, T. (1990) 'Integrating

Children with Severe Disabled Outdoor Education: Focus on Feasibility', *Mental Retardation, 28,* 7-14.

Scroufe, L.A. and Rutter, M. (1984) 'The Domain of Developmental Psychopathology', *Child Development, 55,* 17-29.

Smith, D. (1982) 'Trends in Counseling and Psychotherapy', *American Pscychology, 37,* 802-809.

Smith, E. (1977) 'Counseling Black Individuals: Some Stereotypes', *Personality and Guidance Journal, 55,* 390-397.

Stern, D. (1985) *The Interpersonal World of the Infant,* Basic Books, New York.

Stone, A.A. and Neale, J.M. (1984) 'New Measure of Daily Coping: Development and Preliminary Results', *Journal of Personality and Social Psychology, 46,* 892-906.

Sue, D.W. (1978) 'Counseling Across Cultures', *Personnel and Guidance Journal ,56,* 451.

Sue, D.W. and Sue, D. (1977) 'Barriers to Effective Cross-cultural Counseling', *Journal of Counseling Psychology, 24,* 420-429.

Suelzle, M. and Keenan, V. (1981) 'Changes in Family Support Networks over the Life Cycle of Mentally Retarded Persons', *American Journal of Mental Deficiency, 86,* 267-274.

Sundberg, N.A. (1977) *Assessment of Persons,* Prentice-Hall, Englewood Cliffs, N.J.

Sundberg, N.A., Snowden, L.R. and Reynolds, W.M. (1978) 'Towards Assessment of Personnel Competence and Incompetence in Life Situations', *Annual Review of Psychology, 29,* 179-221.

Thompson, A.P. (1986) 'Changes in Counseling Skills During Undergraduate Study', *Journal of Counseling Psychology, 33,* 65-72.

Tracey, T.J., Hays, K.A., Malone, J. and Herman, B. (1988) 'Changes in Counselor Response as a Function of Experience', *Journal of Counseling Psychology ,35,* 119-126.

Ward, D.E. (1983) 'The Trend Towards Eclecticism and the Development of Comprehensive Models to Guide Counseling and Psychotherapy', *Personnel and Guidance Journal, 62,* 154-157.

Ward, J. (1989) 'Obtaining Generalization Outcome in Developmentally Disabled Persons: A Review of the Current Methodologies', in R.I. Brown and M. Chazan (eds), *Learning Difficulties and Emotional Problems,* Detselig Enterprises Ltd., Calgary.

Weir, E.C. (1965) 'The Meaning of Learning and the Learning of Meaning,' *Phi Delta Kappan, 2,* 280-284.

Whelan, E., Speake, B. and Strickland, T. (1984), 'Action Research: Working with Adult Training Centres in Britain', in R. I. Brown (ed), *Integrated Programmes for Handicapped Adolescents and Adults,* (Vol.1.), Croom Helm, London.

Wikler, L. (1986) 'Periodic Stresses of Families of Older Mentally Retarded Children', *American Journal of Mental Deficiency, 90,* 703-706.

Wode, H. (1983) 'Precursors and the Study of the Impaired Language Learner', in A.E. Mills (ed), *Language Acquisition in the Blind Child: Normal and Deficient,* Croom Helm, London.

Wrenn, C.G. (1976) 'Values and Counseling in Different Countries and Cultures', *The School Counselor, 24,* 6-14.

Wrubel, J., Benner, P. and Lazarus, R.S. (1981) 'Social Competence from the Perspective of Stress and Coping', in J.D. Wine and M.D. Smye (eds), *Social Competence,* The Guilford Press, New York.

Zamble, E. and Porporino, F.J. (1988) *Coping, Behavior and Adaptation in Prison Inmates.,* Springer-Verleg, New York.

Zigler, E. and Glick, M. (1986) *A Developmental Approach to Adult Psychopathology,* John Wiley, New York.

Chapter Six

COUNSELLING ADULTS WITH PHYSICAL DISABILITIES: A TRANSITIONS PERSPECTIVE

Sharon E. Robertson

INTRODUCTION

Over the past 30 years or so, considerable attention has been directed towards how people deal with major life crises especially those associated with physical illness or injury. Based upon Lindemann's (1979) work on the process of grief and mourning and Erikson's (1963) ideas of "developmental crises" at transition points in the life cycle, crisis theory deals with the impact of disruptions on established patterns of personal and social identity. It is postulated that, similar to the need for physiological homeostasis, individuals have a need for social and psychological equilibrium. When a person encounters an event such as a physical illness or injury that upsets his or her characteristic patterns of behaviour and life-style, habitual coping mechanisms are used to restore balance. When a situation is so new or so significant that habitual problem-solving responses are inadequate, a state of disruption or crisis is induced and the individual often experiences unpleasant feelings such as anxiety and guilt (Moos and Tsu, 1976). Such disruptions represent risk because they involve a loss, the threat of such a loss, or a challenge and require that adjustments and adaptations be made. During such crisis periods, an individual may succeed in mastering the distressing experience and emerge stronger and better able to deal effectively in the future, not only with similar stresses, but also with other difficulties as well. Alternatively, he or she may deal with the problems in a maladaptive manner and emerge less healthy than before the crisis began. Whatever the outcome, the new pattern of coping worked out in dealing with the crisis, becomes an integral part of the individual's problem-solving repertoire and increases the chances of dealing more or less realistically with future crises.

Although crisis theory emphasizes the need for new patterns of behaviour, it does not allow for the kinds of life events that often involve gains rather than (or as well as) losses. Furthermore, the term, "crisis" implies a dramatic event, and excludes less observable events and nonevents (Schlossberg, 1984). It also focuses on a relatively brief as opposed to a more extended period of time. Since persons with physical illnesses and disabilities frequently are confronted with many challenges and changes throughout their lifespan in addition to those occurring at the time of injury or onset of an illness, the broader perspective provided by work on life transitions would seem to offer a more comprehensive framework for understanding and counselling persons with physical disabilities.

According to Hopson and Adams (1976), a transition is a personal discontinuity in an individual's life of which he or she is aware and which requires new behavioural responses, because the situation is new and/or the required behaviours are novel. For Schlossberg (1984), a transition is "any event or nonevent that results in change in relationships, routines, assumptions, and/or roles within the settings of self, work, family, health, and/or economics" (p. 43). Such a definition incorporates concepts such as crisis, transformation and change which are frequently used by other authors. For Hopson and Adams (1976) and Schlossberg (1981, 1984), individual perception plays a significant role in defining a transition event. In other words, it is the individual's perception of the change rather than the change event itself that is salient as individuals experience transition events, such as job change, in their own unique ways.

Examples of life transitions include both biological events (e.g., birth, puberty, illness or death of a loved one, personal illness or disability, accident or a surgical operation) and role changes (e.g., entry into school, transfer to high school, leaving school, finding or losing a job, getting married, becoming a parent, becoming divorced, retiring). In fact, some events such as giving birth to a child involve both a biological and a role change. According to Schlossberg (1981, 1984), transitions include not only obvious life changes but also subtle changes (such as the loss of aspirations to marry and the nonoccurrence of anticipated events, such as parenthood). Thus both events and nonevents can be transitions as long as they result in change.

In this chapter, a general transitions framework for understanding psychosocial issues in counselling is presented. The transition process itself is considered in terms of various phases of assimilation followed by a discussion of the influence of cognitive appraisals in affecting individual responses to the transition event. Factors which affect the outcome of the transition process, including those pertaining to the particular transition, the particular environment and the particular individual are outlined. Based upon this framework, specific interventions for counselling persons in transition are suggested. The chapter ends with a summary and recommendations. It is important to note that in this chapter focus is placed primarily on providing a general framework for dealing with various types of life transitions, although specific emphasis is given to the process of responding to a life transition involving physical illness or injury.

THE TRANSITION PROCESS

Transition has been viewed as a process consisting of fairly predictable stages that flow into one another. They often overlap and recycle through earlier stages. Schlossberg (1984) notes that as an individual undergoes a transition, he or she passes through a series of phases (or stages) of assimilation, a process of moving from total preoccupation with the transition to integration of the transition into his or her life.

Beginning with the grieving process model found in the literature on dying (e.g., Kubler-Ross, 1975; Parkes and Weiss, 1983), Hopson and Adams (1977) developed a seven-stage transition process model for life transitions in general. Their stages are related to experienced level of self-esteem. Brammer (1991) has used Hopson's (1981) revised process-stage model which involves six critical points representing the process of movement through time as a framework for his discussion of strategies to use in coping with a life transition. According to this modified model, "the process of adjustment to a transition moves from high personal integration, to disorganization and distress (a downward movement of mood and self-esteem), back up to integration" (Brammer, 1991, p. 23).

A number of theoretical models have been proposed to account for what is believed to be a series of psychosocial phases of adjustment to a physical disability. According to Livneh (1986a), these models tend to differ on three major dimensions:

1. The clinical-theoretical orientation;
2. The nature of the disability (e.g., suddenness of onset, degree of severity, degree of visibility, body part or function affected);
3. The number of stages suggested to account for the variability in adaptation to the disability process.

The different models also address an extensive number of disability-related factors. A number of models deal with crisis-type situations, in which the sudden, traumatic nature of the impairment is prominent (e.g., amputations, myocardial infarction, spinal cord injury). Other models describe stages of adjustment to disabilities having a more gradual onset and progression (e.g., cancer, Huntington's disease, multiple sclerosis). Models also differ in terms of the degree of life-threat associated with the disability (e.g., cancer or myocardial infarction vs. blindness or deafness), the stress placed upon the visibility or cosmetic effect involved (e.g., amputations, spinal cord injury vs. deafness, cardiovascular diseases) and the specific body part(s) or function(s) involved.

Some basic assumptions shared by these stage models include:

1. The onset of a traumatic event has a sudden, unexpected, and tremendously pervasive effect on the individual's life, creating psychological disequilibrium;
2. The adjustment process described applies only to traumas which result in permanent, significant, overt, and perceptually undeniable changes in the body or its function;
3. The process of adaptation is a dynamic and ongoing process consisting of attempts to achieve a new psychological equilibrium;
4. Normal adaptation to the disability involves a temporal sequence of psychosocial developmental stages which seem to be internally triggered and are temporary in nature. However, these stages are not discrete and categorically exclusive; there is overlap among them;
5. The length of time taken to pass through each stage varies across individuals;

6. The process of adaptation to a disability is not irreversible and there is some variability among individuals in their progression through the stages including regression to earlier stages, becoming stuck in certain stages, and skipping or quickly passing through some stages. Furthermore, not all individuals who acquire a disability reach a point of re-integration;
7. Success in responding to the transition produces increased psychosocial growth and maturity;
8. Appropriate external interventions at different points in time, in the form of psychosocial, behavioural, or environmental interventions, may positively affect the coping mechanisms adopted to master the limitations imposed by the disability (Livneh, 1986a).

Based on a review of over 40 stage models of psychosocial adaptation to physical disability, Livneh (1986a) suggested that these models be incorporated into a unified model consisting of five broad stages:

1. Initial impact marked by shock and anxiety;
2. Defense mobilization involving bargaining and denial;
3. Initial realization or recognition involving mourning and/or depression and internalized anger;
4. Retaliation or rebellion marked by both direct and indirect methods of externalizing anger and aggressiveness;
5. Reintegration or reorganization involving cognitive (acknowledgement), affective (acceptance) and behavioural (final adjustment or reconstruction) dimensions.

Each of the suggested stages is further described in terms of the typical defense mechanisms used, the types of emotions experienced, the associated thought processes operating, the observed activities engaged in and the direction (internal or external) of the energy expended. This model has much in common with the Hopson (1981) model referred to previously.

According to Brammer (1991), models such as this are useful in helping individuals make sense out of their transitions and in putting their feelings into words. However, they must be used cautiously since there is limited evidence for a stage process model. In addition, it should be noted that one does not automatically pass through these stages in a mechanical fashion. Various factors are believed to mediate the process of change including the nature of the transition event, the environment, and the individual's personal characteristics and coping resources. Furthermore, the individual's reactions are linked to his or her continuous and changing appraisal of him or herself in the situation at that time.

COGNITIVE APPRAISAL

According to Lazarus and Folkman (1984), appraisal consists of a continuously changing set of judgments about the significance of events to personal well-being and it is the central component of an individual's self-regulating system. Appraisal involves perceiving distinctions between potentially harmful, promising and irrelevant aspects of the environment. A person may then appraise the personal and social demands of a situation and judge how to act, based on his or her perceived power to master the environment's demands (Brammer and Abrego, 1981).

The appraisal process is categorized by Lazarus into primary appraisal, secondary appraisal and reappraisal. Although it might appear that these processes occur sequentially, this is not so. In fact, the two processes may occur simultaneously, differing in function and not in timing. Primary appraisal involves an initial judgment that the outcome of a situation will be either beneficial, harmful or irrelevant. Appraisal of a situation as beneficial means that the person believes that no coping efforts are required. However, it may be combined with a mild threat over the possibility of its loss. Appraisals that arouse stress may relate to harm or loss that has already occurred, threat of harm or loss or challenge. If a situation is appraised as irrelevant, it is not considered to have any threatening or beneficial implications for personal well being. In addition to the primary appraisal of whether a transition is positive, stressful or irrelevant, individuals make a secondary appraisal (i.e., an appraisal of their coping resources which include themselves, their supports and their options). As an individual considers various alternatives for dealing with threats or loss, his or her coping responses are formulated and modified. Furthermore, through this secondary appraisal process, an initial primary appraisal of a situation may be changed. For example, in considering coping responses, a person may begin to feel that he or she can overcome a threat resulting in a reduction in the initial appraisal of harm. Reappraisal involves altering one's original perception of events in response to changing external or internal conditions and results in re-evaluation of decisions based on feedback from a changing environment. Individual reactions associated with cognitive appraisals are more complex than they might appear. Dealing with threat involves both cognitive and emotional processes as threat arouses various feelings which affect the physiological level of arousal. The individual's own appraisal and reappraisal of the transition, the basic adaptive tasks required, his or her resources for coping, and the results of coping efforts play a critical role in the transition process.

OTHER VARIABLES AFFECTING OUTCOME

The individual's cognitive appraisal, definition of the adaptive tasks involved, and selection and effectiveness of coping skills are influenced by three sets of variables:

1. Characteristics of the transition;
2. Characteristics of the environment;
3. Characteristics of the individual.

These factors jointly affect the initial resolution of the transition and it, in turn, alters them, thereby changing the ultimate outcome. Each of these is discussed in more detail.

Transition Characteristics

A number of variables have been postulated to characterize transitions in general, and to affect the coping process and ultimately the outcome for the individual (Schlossberg, 1981, 1984). These include the type of transition (anticipated, unanticipated, chronic hassle, nonevent), the context in which it occurs, the impact, the trigger (precipitator), the timing (on-time or off-time), the source (internal or external), role change (gain or loss), duration (permanent, temporary, or uncertain), previous experience with a similar transition and concurrent stress. Consideration is given to each of these within the following section.

Types of transition. According to Hopson and Adams (1976), transitions may be categorized according to size ranging from macro-transitions like war, earthquakes or technological change, to micro-transitions at the individual level relating to a person's marriage, career and relationships. They can also be categorized according to the degree to which they are predictable and voluntary.

Predictable or anticipated transitions result from normative changes of a major nature in roles that occur in the course of an individual's life. Their onset is usually gradual. These expected events include, for example, leaving home and marrying. In terms of health, a person may have a life-long expectation of illness because of family history. For example, a father may have died of a heart attack at a relatively early age or a number of family members may have died of cancer. Because these are events that are likely to occur, one can anticipate and rehearse or prepare for them.

Unpredictable or unanticipated transitions are unscheduled events that are unexpected. These usually "involve crises, eruptive circumstances, and other unexpected occurrences that are not the consequence of life-cycle transitions" (Pearlin, 1980, p.179). Their onset is usually sudden. As no preparation or rehearsal is possible with these transitions, they are usually more difficult to assimilate than those that are expected. Events of this type in the health sphere include, for example, unexpected illness or injury. Moreover, the cue to action may not be an illness event but a diagnosis of risk for chronic illness or increased disability (Loveys, 1990). In the vocational area, they include, for example, being laid off or being promoted. In the marital arena, they include divorce and premature death of a spouse. It is important to note that what is an anticipated change for one person (e.g., leaving work) might be unanticipated for another.

In addition to the predictable and unpredictable

transitions identified by Hopson and Adams (1976), Schlossberg (1984) adds two categories of transitions: chronic hassles and nonevents. Transitions involving chronic hassles are characterized by their continuous and pervasive presence. Some persistent hassles include concern with weight, health of a family member, upkeep of property and transportation (Lazarus and Folkman, 1984). These chronic hassles can erode self-confidence and lead to an inability to initiate necessary changes. A major life event such as diagnosis of chronic illness would fall into this category. In addition to its obvious or immediate impact, it can create continuing hassles.

Nonevent transitions are those an individual had expected but which did not occur. In some cases such nonevent transitions may be more stressful or may be perceived to be more stressful than the transition involved if the event had occurred. Moreover, a nonevent for one person (e.g., not having children) can be a planned decision for someone else and therefore, not a transition at all .

Transitions may be further characterized according to the events with which they are associated (e.g., marriage, divorce, illness). According to Moos and Schaefer (1984), factors which must be considered in illness-related transitions include the type and location of symptoms-whether painful, disfiguring, disabling or in a body region vested with special importance such as the heart or reproductive organs. These factors are a major component in defining the exact nature of the tasks patients and others face, and consequently, their adaptive responses. Different body parts and functions may have a psychological significance that has little to do with biological factors related to survival. For example, a facial injury or a breast amputation may have a stronger psychological impact on a woman than severe hypertension which directly threatens her life.

Context. The context in which a transition event occurs may influence how that event is perceived and how a person responds to it. One can try to understand the context by looking at the relationship of the person to the transition (Schlossberg, 1984). A transition may be centred within the person, in an interpersonal relationship, or within the community. One might also look at the setting within which the transition is taking place: self, family, friends, work, health or finances. So, for example, within the health setting (AIDS), a transition may begin with the individual's own illness, with his or her spouse's illness or with public attitudes and policies toward the illness. Also, within the context of personal health, the transition of an individual who has not been in a sick role (i.e., has been healthy and diagnosed at risk for illness) will differ from an individual who is moving from an illness episode to a chronic condition (Loveys, 1990).

Impact. The impact of a transition event can be assessed by examining the degree to which a person's daily life is changed. In effect, with greater degrees of change, more coping resources are needed and a longer time may be taken to assimilate the experience into a modified lifestyle. According to Cohen and Lazarus (1979), almost all serious illnesses threaten the individual to some extent. The imposed threats usually consist of threats to life itself, threats to bodily integrity and comfort, threats to self-concept and future plans, threats to emotional equilibrium and threats to the accomplishment of customary roles and social activities. There are also the threats associated with the need to adjust to a new physical or social environment. While different types of illnesses and medical interventions arouse similar threats and similar needs for adjustment, they may vary in terms of the degree of impact and the types of coping strategies required because of the nature of the disease involved. For the person who is diagnosed as being at-risk for further illness, the impact of this transition may not be readily obvious to others although the uncertainty and ambiguity associated with this situation may contribute to a heightened sense of vulnerability for the individual affected (Loveys, 1990).

The impact of a transition will usually diminish over time. For the person with a chronic illness, it is probable that the more time that passes without a relapse, the less impact the transition event will have on the perceived potential for risk (Loveys, 1990).

Trigger. A transition is usually set off by a specific event that makes the individual look at his or her life differently at a particular point in time. What triggers a transition varies from person to person. For the person who becomes disabled in midlife, the trigger is the onset of disability (Power, Hershenson and Schlossberg, 1985). For the spouse of a person who, for example, has had a heart attack or cancer, the trigger for a midlife transition may be body changes in one's partner.

Timing. Most adults expect certain life events to occur within particular periods of time and they judge whether they are "on time" or "off time" accordingly. Normative transitions such as having children or enrolling in post-secondary education are usually linked in people's minds with a certain age. To be off time, whether early or late, often carries negative social and psychological consequences. An example of an off-time transition would be involuntary retirement at 35. The death of a child or young adult would be considered an off-time event, whereas the death of an elderly parent would be considered on-time. For the person who acquires a disability, the timing of this transition is almost never on schedule. Indeed, it may exacerbate the impact of a normal developmental transition if the two events occur simultaneously (Myers, 1985) .

Source. An individual's perceived control or mastery in a situation   affects the degree to which events are perceived as threatening (Lazarus and Launier, 1978). The source of some transitions is internal (i.e., voluntary), a deliberate decision on the part of the individual, whereas the source of others is completely external (i.e., involuntary) and the transition is forced upon the individual by other people or by circumstances. For most adults, disability represents an unwelcome transition and the source is almost always beyond the individual's control as in an injury arising from an automobile accident or in the development of a brain tumour. Individuals generally assimilate voluntary transitions more easily than involuntary ones because of the degree of personal control perceived to be exercised. Thus the person who quits a job voluntarily probably finds the change less threatening than the person who is fired or leaves because of ill health.

Role Change. According to role theory, roles consist of socially defined behavioural expectations for individuals occupying certain positions and for those who interact with them. Most transitions are accompanied by changes in roles involving gains (e.g., getting promoted, getting married, becoming a parent) and/or losses (e.g., becoming widowed, getting divorced, retiring). Furthermore, role change can be more or less difficult (and have greater or lesser impact) depending on whether the new role involves primarily a loss or a gain, is positive or negative or has explicit norms and expectations for the person assuming it. Nevertheless, regardless of whether a transition predominantly involves a role gain or loss, it will be accompanied by various expectations and accompanying anxiety. The more an individual engages in "anticipatory socialization", orientation toward the values and norms of the new role, the sooner that he or she will be comfortable.

The person who is hospitalized is expected to assume the patient or sick role although this may be contrary to his or her wishes. Often patients wish to maintain as much authority and control as possible. As the individual moves from the hospital back to the home, the role expectations of the health care professionals will be replaced by the role expectations of the person's family and friends. Personal and societal expectations for the roles to be assumed will also influence whether an individual perceives that any given role can be abandoned (Loveys, 1990). A conflict in role expectations may occur as a person returns to his or her daily routines following an illness while family members continue to attend to the illness. For example, a heart attack survivor may undertake to follow an exercise regimen which is beneficial for his or her recovery while family members may try to keep him or her in the role of an ill person by encouraging sedentary behaviours. The reverse may also occur; a family may expect a heart attack survivor who has no obvious disability to resume daily living patterns (including high-risk diets, etc.) while the individual remains in a patient role and wants comfort and support.

Duration. Another variable which affects the ease or difficulty of assimilating the transition is its expected duration (i.e., whether it is expected to be permanent or temporary). A transition that is painful and unpleasant may be more easily borne if the individual is assured that it is of limited duration, as when someone enters the hospital for surgery that he or she knows will be minor and will have no lasting effects. However, there are situations in which such expectations are not fulfilled and the individual's condition is found to be more serious than predicted (e.g., a malignant tumour). In such circumstances, the person is likely to have more difficulty in assimilating the transition. Conversely, if the change is desired, then the certainty that it represents a more or less permanent state may be reassuring.

Uncertainty is connected with perhaps the greatest degree of stress and negative affect. Illness seems to imply uncertainty. Uncertainty and ambiguity pervade chronic illness and can be highly anxiety-provoking. The uncertainty experienced by the person with a chronic illness is related to an inability to attach definite meaning to the illness experience: the possibility of progression or recurrence of the illness is uncertain, experienced symptoms may be ominous or of no consequence, and the relative effectiveness of recommended treatments and health-promoting behaviours is unclear (Loveys, 1990).

Previous Experience with a Similar Transition. The individual who has successfully weathered a particular kind of transition in the past will probably be successful at assimilating another transition of a similar nature. Conversely, the person who has been defeated by a situation may become more vulnerable and less able to cope in the future. Past experiences to some extent determine the person's mental set, and if that past experience was unfavourable, then the mental set may be something of a self-fulfilling prophecy. For individuals who acquire disabilities, the degree of previous similar experience will vary from person to person.

One of the expected outcomes from experiencing a life transition is to develop a way of thinking about life transitions. This act of conceptualization may reduce fear of future transitions by giving a measure of predictability to and understanding of the change events (Brammer, 1991).

Concurrent Stress. The greater the number of other simultaneous transitions, the harder it will be for the person to cope with any one of them. So, for the individual who acquires disabilities, the more concurrent stress, the more difficult it will be to cope with transition to a life style involving disability. A person who, in rapid sequence, gets divorced, loses a job and suffers a heart attack is likely to have a harder time than will the person who acquires a disability but can maintain a marriage and return to a job (Power *et al.*, 1985). In fact, often transitions in one area stimulate other stresses and transitions. For example, the person who has suffered from spinal cord injury may find that he or she must give up a job. Being unemployed brings with it its own stresses including financial problems as well as lack of structure and meaning in one's life. This situation may further precipitate marital and relationship problems which result in divorce. The stressfulness of a particular event depends not so much on the event itself as on the balance between a person's liabilities and assets at the time the event occurs.

Environmental Characteristics

Both the physical and psychosocial environment influence how a person responds to and deals with a transition. Each of these is considered further.

Physical Environment. Characteristics of the physical environment include the aesthetic quality of one's environment and the amount of personal space available (Brammer and Abrego, 1981). Considering illness-related transitions, Moos and Schaefer (1984) state, "the physical features of a hospital, or of special areas such as intensive care units, with their unfamiliar sights and sounds and bustle of activity, can further upset patients already burdened by a painful illness" (p. 21). Other features of the physical environment such as the availability of wheelchairs for the elderly in shopping malls and ramps for wheelchairs in buildings and on curbs are sensitive changes that lessen handicaps. The designation of certain days as "Disability Days" for shopping at a particular store may make the physical environment more or less manageable but may add negatively to a self perception of disability and incompetence. What is of assistance to some may be viewed negatively by others.

Psychosocial Environment. The psychosocial environment includes the range of individuals with whom one relates during transitions whether they are part of intimate relationships, family units, networks of friends, institutions or communities. Counsellors, rehabilitation personnel, medical staff and members of the clergy and social service agencies are examples of the professional network. According to Lazarus and Launier (1978), the knowledge of existing or available support, either actual or imagined, affects an individual's perception of stress and his or her assessment of his or her capacity to cope with threats.

Gottlieb (1983) states that "social support consists of verbal and/or nonverbal information or advice, tangible aid, or action that is proffered by social intimates or inferred by their presence and has beneficial behavioural effects on the recipient" (p.28). Most commonly, social support consists of a number of interrelated types:

1. Emotional support or esteem support;
2. Instrumental support or tangible aid and services;
3. Informational support or cognitive guidance;
4. Social companionship.

Implicit in most conceptualizations of social support is the idea that one is part of a reliable alliance in which there is a genuine concern for one's well-being and in which certain people and resources are available, if needed.

No single network is suitable for all stages of the lifespan; rather networks of differing size, density and composition appear to be appropriate in differing situations. There is a growing body of evidence linking isolation or a lack of confiding relationships with various forms of psychopathology. Further, various factors (e.g., long-term illness) may tend to diminish network size, although the quality of support can remain high. Various types of structural forms may be differentially appropriate throughout the life span. In times of loss, a dense, emotionally supportive network may be most satisfying, while in times of re-orientation, a loosely-knit structure of relationships with more variety and far-reaching ties may be more adaptive. Neighbours and friends are usually relied on for services, emergencies and short-term difficulties while relatives are sources of financial and long-term assistance. Types of social support vary not only within the specific challenge an individual faces, but also with the stage within the particular transition period (Saulnier, 1982). Wesolowski (1987) reported that vocational rehabilitation clients had significantly smaller social networks than non-clients, that the type of disability had no effect on the size of social networks and that the sizes of networks decreased with age among clients whereas they increased with age with non-clients.

The value of social support as a means of decreasing vulnerability to physical disease and disability and of facilitating recovery from various illnesses has been the subject of study for some time. For example, Doehrman (1977), Gottlieb (1983) and Kaplan and Toshima (1990) reviewed work on cardiac patients; Dushensko (1981), Hymovich and Baker (1985) and Patterson (1985) reported on cystic fibrosis; and Gottlieb (1983) and Ingram (1989) focused on breast cancer. It has been suggested that family, friends and other social contacts can ease the emotional stress resulting from injuries incurred in automobile accidents (Porritt, 1979); that burn victims experience higher self-esteem and general life satisfaction if they have support from friends and family (Davidson, Bowden, and Tholen, 1979); that patients with kidney disease who have support from spouses and cohesive families have a higher morale and fewer changes in social functioning during haemodialysis than do those with less support (Dimond, 1979); and that males have better outcomes following myocardial infarction if they have support from their spouses (Finlayson, 1976). In a similar vein, Kaplan and Toshima (1990) explored the complex relationships among adaptations to chronic illness, self-care and the social environment with respect to specific chronic illnesses (non-insulin-dependent diabetes mellitus, coronary heart disease and back pain). Following an extensive review of studies in this area, they reported that caring family members may have a positive effect on health outcomes but only if they reinforce appropriate health behaviours. Without reviewing the literature in detail, suffice it to say that many studies suggest a social support-health outcome connection. In fact, according to Moos and Schaefer (1984), "The course of an illness tends to be more benign, and recovery tends to be quicker than expected, when it occurs in the context of interpersonal understanding and empathy" (p. 21).

Following an extensive examination of studies of social support to assess its impact in promoting recovery from acute illness and coping with serious physical illness and injury such as asthma, hypertension, stroke, coronary disease and myocardial infarction, cancer, mastectomy and orthopaedic disability, Di Matteo and Hays (1981) outlined specific potential beneficial effects of social support in recovering from serious illness or injury. Tangible social support such as financial help, running errands, and child care tend to be highly valued when one is ill. Tangible social support may help to reduce the ill person's pain, tiredness and worry and may also make it easier to comply with therapeutic regimens. Reactions of others may help the ill person assess the threatening quality of a situation and to gauge his or her own level of arousal. People with physical illnesses or disfigurements in particular look to others for validation of their own personal value and worth and for feedback about their behaviour thereby affecting self-image and self-esteem. The social network may also provide an opportunity to discuss feelings, express emotions and develop intimacy during times of illness. Further, those who are close to the person with a disability may have the most influence in changing his or her attitudes and behaviours particularly as it relates to compliance with medical regimens that require a difficult change and the adoption of appropriate health behaviours. Members of the support environment may model appropriate coping skills and health behaviours (Pearlin and Aneshensel, 1986). Thus, if a network member makes health-promoting changes at the same time as the person with the disability, the outcome may be enhanced through mutual encouragement, mutual modelling and a reduction in the perceived difficulty of making the changes. Adaptation may be made easier by having network members absorb some of the stress (Kaplan and Toshima, 1990).

In some circumstances, social networks can have a detrimental effect on individuals and this is no less true in the case of recovery from physical illness (Coyne, Wortman and

Lehman, 1988). Various aspects of a possible miscarried helping process have been discussed in the context of chronic pain (Maruta, Osbourne, Swanson and Hallnig, 1981), disability (Fengler and Goodrich, 1979), and illness, such as Alzheimer's disease (Ware and Carper, 1982), renal failure (Malmquist and Hagberg, 1974) and stroke (Watzlawick and Coyne, 1980). Serious illness or injury to one family member can put undue stress on the others resulting in negative effects on the family equilibrium (Di Matteo and Hays, 1981; Hymovich and Baker, 1985; Patterson, 1985; Vargo, 1979). If the person with the disability receives too much attention, the resources of the other members of the family system may gradually become depleted leading to chronic illness and symptoms, frustrations and interpersonal conflict. The person with a disability may be distressed by the "burden" (emotional, physical, financial) that he or she places on others. Members may become disengaged from one another with the accompanying destruction of emotional bonds, if issues of equity and reciprocity of support are not dealt with. The person with a disability must learn how he or she can offer support to others. Coyne *et al.*, (1988) identify the following ways in which family members' emotional over-involvement in being helpful can prove self-defeating. First, it may simply interfere with their problem-solving or performance of instrumental tasks; Second, emotionally over-involved family members may become too focused on the instrumental outcomes of their helping efforts or demonstrations of their helpfulness to be aware that they are communicating to the recipient in ways which leave the recipient feeling guilty, incompetent, resentful, lacking in autonomy or coerced; Third, over time the helper and recipient may accumulate issues (e.g, about who's in control in their relationship) that take precedence over other concerns (e.g., compliance with the treatment regimen).

On a broader level, Schweitzer (1982) and Vargo (1989) comment on the role of the media as well as health care professionals in promoting attitudes which are stigmatizing toward persons with disabilities. The media traditionally have characterized persons with physical disabilities as maladjusted, infirm, pathetic and yet courageous superstars, while treatment of medical problems familiarizes the person who has a disability with the role of the sick person entailing passivity, dependency and submission to treatment. The stigma experienced on a daily basis by many individuals with disabilities, primarily when interacting with able-bodied individuals who are uncomfortable with the person's disability, can affect the self-concept, sense of body image and group identification and acquisition of coping skills. Frequently, a perceiver has a negative association to one aspect of an individual (the impairment) and generalizes this association to other aspects of the individual such as his or her character or intelligence. Such negative attitudes may become incorporated into the self-concept of the person with the disability.

Individual Characteristics

A number of personality and background factors influence the range of coping responses that an individual perceives to be available in a given situation (Brammer and Abrego, 1981). As Schlossberg (1981, 1984) notes, these factors include socioeconomic status, sex role, age and stage of life, state of health, ego development, personality, cultural background, commitments and values and coping responses. According to Moos and Schaefer (1984), similar factors influence the individual's appraisal of an illness and affect the personal and social resources available to meet the crisis. Several of these factors are discussed in more detail.

Age and Life Stage. Chronological age is relatively unimportant compared to one's capacity to respond to societal pressures and required tasks to participate in roles assigned by society and to function or perform as expected of people in one's age brackets (Schlossberg, 1984). Hence, the timing of an illness or a disability in the life cycle is particularly important. For example, a child who has become an invalid because of rheumatic heart disease has different concerns than does an elderly patient who has been incapacitated by a heart ailment (Moos and Schaefer, 1984). Some adolescents have a hard time coping with physical illness because it imposes an added stress just when the young person is faced with the challenging psychosocial tasks of adolescence which include adjusting to the physical and physiological changes of puberty, establishing effective social and working relationships with the same- and opposite-sex peers, achieving independence from primary caretakers, preparing for a vocation and moving toward a sense of values and a sense of definable identity (Davis, Anderson, Linkowski, Berger and Feinstein, 1985). According to Power *et al.*, (1985), middle age is a period of high risk for both sexes in that they are more likely to experience negative rather than positive stresses and to be overwhelmed by them. They propose that those individuals who must confront the transition to disability in midlife, either because it occurs at that time or because it is brought into that period unresolved from earlier in life, are at special risk in dealing with the other transitions that typically accompany the middle years, such as changes in sexuality and in family and work roles. Issues such as the threatened disruption of established roles and the lack of fulfilment of cherished life aims which are important for individuals in midlife who are confronted with a disability may be less salient for the elderly, but elderly persons often suffer from some cognitive impairment that reduces their coping ability.

State of Health. The individual's state of health not only affects his or her ability to assimilate a transition but also may itself be a source of stress which precipitates a transition. In some cases, a person may recover quickly from an acute but minor illness and be left relatively unaffected, with little change in self-perception. In other cases, an illness, though short, may remind the person of his or her own mortality and thus have lasting psychological effects. In still other cases, the illness may be chronic, leading to a gradual decline in physical resources and energy level and thus severely affecting the individual's ability to cope (Power *et al.*, 1985).

Personality. Self-esteem and mastery have been identified as two major psychological variables affecting an individual's response to a transition. Self-esteem refers to an individual's evaluation of the self, whether positive or negative. Awareness of physical changes may affect self-esteem which in turn affects personal goals. The enforced dependency and passivity associated with illness is especially likely to be problematic for individuals who pride themselves on being assertive and independent (Moos and Schaefer, 1984).

Mastery, like locus of control, refers to an individual's ability to be in charge of his or her life (Pearlin and Schooler, 1978). In addition to mediating one's assessment of the severity of stress, this expectancy of control affects one's awareness of available coping alternatives. To the extent that people judge themselves to have control in a situation, the probability is that they will be less likely to perceive the situation as threatening and, in turn, less likely to manifest adverse reaction patterns (Lazarus and Launier, 1978). Brammer and Abrego (1981) refer to Abramson, Seligman and Teasdale's (1978) and Seligman's (1975) theory of learned helplessness as having important implications for understanding the individual in transition. According to this theory, "when an individual's efforts to cope with a problematic situation are perceived as being reinforced on a non-contingent basis, and an individual becomes aware of present and past non-contingencies, he or she develops an internal attribution for why consequences are independent of his or her emitted responses. These attributions lead to a negative expectancy about the future, experience of helplessness, and behavioural signs of depression. Learned helplessness becomes manifested in motivational, cognitive, self-esteem, and affective deficiencies " (p. 23). Thus, the two sources of control, internal and external, interact. The degree to which the trigger or transition is in or out of the individual's control and the degree to which the individual can control his or her reactions to it are important in characterizing transitions.

Cultural Background. Culture forms the context in which stressful life events derive their meaning. Each culture has its own yardstick for measuring the stressfulness of any life event so that, in effect, what is viewed as stressful in one culture may not be viewed as stressful in another (Smith, 1985). For example, in Western societies, retirement often is considered as the end of one's productivity and becomes associated with lowered social status. In some third world societies, transition out of the work force is valued and results in higher social status (Brammer and Abrego, 1981).

Vargo (1989) points out that people who are visibly different are more openly accepted in some cultures than in others, with generally more acceptance shown in highly industrialized countries. As pointed out earlier, the greater nonacceptance of individuals with disability within one's culture, the more difficult the adjustment to disability is likely to be. One source of nonacceptance of individuals with disabilities in Judeao-Christian cultures is long standing religious beliefs wherein physical and mental disorders are viewed as punishments inflicted by God for past wrongdoings. If one adheres to this perspective, then one is likely to feel guilt, remorse and sinfulness which would impede the process of adaptation to disability. In contrast to this is the view that disability is an unfortunate accident or a quirk of fate (Vargo, 1989).

Of particular relevance in the area of rehabilitation is the fact that cultures differ in terms of what they identify as being a disability. What may be a disability in one culture may not be considered to be particularly troublesome or disabling in another. Cultural beliefs about sources of disabling conditions may also affect both the recognition of special needs and the response to offered services. For example, if a disability is seen to arise from family problems, the family may feel responsible for taking care of the person with the disability and keep the individual out of sight so as not to expose their shame to others. In some societies, such as the United States, mild vision impairment is considered to be normal and the wearing of a prosthesis to correct this impairment, attractive. In other societies, the wearing of any prothesis device is ridiculed (Heath and Levin, 1991).

Commitments and Values. An individual's major commitment - whether it is his or her relationships (interpersonal), working for others (altruism), self-improvement (competence/mastery) or survival (self-protective) - determines his or her vulnerability. The husband in a childless marriage, which had lasted 30 years, explained how he had a much more difficult time in making an adjustment to divorce than his wife. Although both were retired, the wife not only initiated the divorce but also had commitments to her own family of origin and her friends which sustained her through the transition process. The husband, on the other hand, had made a major commitment to his wife and his work throughout his adult life. With both gone, he struggled to find meaning in his life. Clearly the reaction to and assimilation of transitions is greatly influenced by commitments which do change over time and, in effect, alter areas of vulnerability.

An individual's basic values and beliefs are also a factor in his or her ability to assimilate transitions. Values which facilitate assimilation of a transition at one stage of life may hinder this process at another (Schlossberg, 1984). Religious beliefs are an obvious example of value orientation that is often said to sustain people through the trials of life. For instance, grief over the death of a loved one may be eased by the belief that the death is "God's will." The specific content of an individual's religious beliefs, and the cultural norms associated with a particular religion, need to be considered also. For example, a woman from a Catholic background facing an abortion may find her distress exacerbated by the church's strictures against such a practice.

Coping Responses. Concurrent with appraising and reappraising events, resources, and results during a transition, an individual engages in coping behaviour. Coping has been defined as the "constantly changing cognitive and behavioural efforts to manage specific external and/or internal demands that are appraised as taxing or exceeding the resources of the person" (Lazarus and Folkman, 1984, p.141). It has also been referred to as "the things people do to avoid being harmed by life strains" (Pearlin and Schooler, 1978, p.1).

Brammer and Abrego (1981) point out several aspects of these definitions of coping which are important:

1. Coping is an emotional rather than a purely cognitive process;
2. Coping may refer to positive stress which is related to promise and opportunity as well as to the distress which results from threat or loss;
3. Coping involves adaptive tasks in which the outcome is uncertain and the limits of the person's adaptive skills are approached.

155

Moos and Tsu (1976) identify four categories of general adaptive tasks which apply to all life crises or transitions. These include preserving a reasonable emotional balance, preserving a satisfactory self-image and maintaining a sense of competence and mastery, sustaining relationships with family and friends and preparing for an uncertain future. They further identify three tasks which are primarily illness related. These include dealing with pain, incapacitation, and other symptoms; dealing with the hospital environment and special treatment procedures and developing and maintaining adequate relationships with health care staff. These seven groups of tasks are generally encountered with every illness, but their relative importance varies, depending on the nature of the disease, the personality of the individual involved and the unique set of circumstances. Similarly, general and specific adaptive tasks exist for other types of transitions (e.g., see Ahrons, 1980; Borgen, Amundson and Biela, 1987; Davis *et al.*, 1985; Kivnick, 1985; Power *et al.*, 1985). These tasks may be as difficult and challenging for family members as for the individual. An individual's assessment of stress, therefore, is based on his or her evaluation of available coping resources in relation to internal or environmental demands.

Most theoretical frameworks describe the coping process as a complex interaction between an individual and the environment. Lazarus and Launier (1978) believe that this interaction is characterized by a "reciprocity of causation." Both the person and the situation impact each other mutually. An individual subjectively appraises threat or promise in the situation by considering personal transition characteristics as well as physical and social environmental factors. As a person directs a coping response to environmental demands, the actual or perceived nature of the environment undergoes change. Environmental demands will change over time in a response to coping efforts and factors associated with the transition itself. A wide range of personality characteristics also affects this appraisal process (Brammer and Abrego, 1981).

Pearlin and Schooler (1978) have identified three types of coping responses:

1. Those that modify the situation (e.g., negotiating, taking optimistic action, seeking advice and exercising potency as opposed to helpless resignation);
2. Those that control the meaning of a stressful experience in

order cognitively to neutralize the threat (e.g., making positive comparisons, selectively ignoring, substituting rewards);
3. Those that function primarily to control emotional distress (e.g., discharging emotions by ventilating feelings, asserting oneself and exercising passive forbearance).

Similarly, Lazarus and Folkman (1984) identify two major coping orientations: instrumental behaviour to change the situation and palliative behaviour to help minimize individual distress. In order to change the situation or reduce personal distress, one can choose from among four coping modes (direct action, inhibition of action, information seeking and intra-psychic [i.e., thoughts such as denial, wishful thinking and distortion, which an individual uses to resolve the issue]).

Schlossberg (1984) has integrated these two models by categorizing coping responses as:

1. Functions;
2. Strategies;

The functions of coping responses are:

1. To control the situation;
2. To control the meaning of it;
3. To control the stress associated with it.

Coping strategies consist of:

1. Information seeking (i.e., seeking advice vs. self-reliance, searching for resources, reading/watching television);
2. Direct action (i.e., negotiation, discipline, emotional discharge, self-assertion, stress management, optimistic action, potency vs. hopeless resignation);
3. Inhibition of action (i.e., selective ignoring, controlled reflection, denial, positive comparisons, substitution of rewards).

Brammer and Abrego (1981) suggest some additional strategies which might be used to reduce anxiety including using drugs, relaxing muscles, averting attention or leaving the situation physically. These strategies to minimize personal discomforts may be necessary before more effective problem-solving may occur.

Effective coping involves flexible use of a range of strategies as each situation demands, and the highly adaptive individual is able to choose those coping responses likely to be most effective in a given situation. Lazarus and Folkman (1984) emphasize the fact that selection of a coping strategy depends on personal dispositions, situations, and available responses. Most theorists see direct action as the preferred mode of coping. However, Lazarus and Folkman (1984) suggest that effective copers use both direct actions and palliative coping modes. Brammer and Abrego (1981) suggest that to become effective, direct action strategies require an awareness of the problematic nature of a situation as well as the knowledge of how to modify it. A person may be too inhibited to try to modify the situation. Also, some situations, such as terminal illness, seem impervious to direct action methods although some action methods directed at modifying the immune system offer some terminally ill individuals hope of influencing the course of their illness (Simonton and Simonton, 1975). Although styles of coping may be effective across a variety of transitions and age spans, some coping skills seem to be particularly effective for specific age groups. For example, Lieberman (1975) has suggested that "combativeness" may be an important coping response for older people.

Individuals in transition need flexible coping options for tolerating or overcoming threats and challenges. Brammer and Abrego (1981) developed a taxonomy of coping skills which seem useful across a variety of transitions. The taxonomy consists of five broad categories of skills and is based upon empirical investigation of the coping process. The first group includes skills in perceiving and responding to transitions. Two important perceptions toward change (i.e., that acceptance of problematic situations are a normal part of living and that each person has a variety of strengths which can help him or her to cope with most situations effectively) affect how a person interprets events. If the individual holds these beliefs, he or she has an increased sense of self control and self esteem, does not feel overwhelmed by change and will attempt to respond to change in an effective way. Other important skills include being able to describe threats accurately, to recognize the role of feelings in appraisal and to inhibit both impulsivity and passivity. These skills in responding to transitions allow individuals to gain awareness of how they think, feel and behave when confronted with a problematic situation. The second group includes skills for assessing, building and using external support systems. Individuals in transition often need extra sources of social support during the times of transition. Skills required in developing and strengthening external social support involve identifying one's emotional needs, identifying people in one's life who provide support, seeking specific people to serve in one's support network and improving the supportive quality of relationships. For those who lack a support network, the skills involve locating and participating in a formalized group. The third group includes skills for assessing, developing and using internal support systems (i.e., self messages or self-talk). Skills in internal support involve restructuring inappropriate self-criticism into supportive self-talk which then can help an individual cope with difficult situations. The fourth group includes skills for reducing emotional and physiological distress through self-relaxation, strategies for controlling too much or too little stimulation and verbal expression of feelings. The fifth and final group includes skills for planning and implementing change including goal setting, decision-making, problem solving, anxiety management and self-assertion.

According to Moos and Schaefer (1984), the most common coping skills used to deal with physical illness can be organized into three domains, according to their primary focus:

1. Appraisal-focused coping;
2. Problem-focused coping;
3. Emotion-focused coping.

Such skills are seldom used singly or exclusively. Appraisal-focused coping involves attempts to understand and find a pattern of meaning in a crisis. This can involve logical analysis of the situation and mentally rehearsing alternative actions and their probable consequences. It also covers cognitive strategies by which an individual accepts the basic reality of a situation but restructures it to find something favourable (cognitive redefinition) as well as an array of skills aimed at denying or minimizing the seriousness of a crisis (cognitive avoidance or denial). Problem-focused coping seeks to confront the reality of a crisis by dealing with its tangible consequences and trying to construct a more satisfying situation. It includes strategies for seeking information and support, taking problem-solving action and identifying alternative rewards. Emotion-focused coping involves controlling the emotions provoked by a distressing situation, discharging or venting one's feelings to reduce tension and/or coming to terms with a situation and accepting it as it is. A health crisis typically presents a variety of related tasks and requires a combination or sequence of coping skills.

Brammer and Abrego (1981) and Brammer (1991) conclude that coping skills can be classified several ways, but a meaningful and simple grouping is appraising potential danger, building support (network, family, friends), restructuring cognitions, managing stressors and solving problems. These skills may be used individually, consecutively or in various combinations. Specific coping strategies are not inherently adaptive or maladaptive. Skills that are effective in one situation may not be in another. Skills that may be beneficial given moderate or temporary use may be harmful if relied upon exclusively. Brammer and Abrego (1981) believe that knowledge of coping skills can be useful in formulating therapeutic interventions, in designing groups for persons in transition and in providing consultation to self-help groups.

INTERVENTION

"The heart of the therapeutic process is the relationship established between counsellor and client" (Brammer and Shostrom, 1977, p.149). Various authors including Egan (1986) have developed models to help counsellors acquire the skills necessary to develop a constructive counselling relationship. Egan (1975) divided the counselling process into three phases (Exploration, Understanding and Action) and identified the counselling skills appropriate to each.

Beginning with Egan's (1975) model, Schlossberg (1984) constructed a generic framework for counselling individuals in transition and divided the counselling process into three sequential phases with the corresponding goals of counselling being:

1. To explore the problem;
2. To facilitate understanding of the problem;
3. To promote coping.

In the first or Exploration phase, the counsellor's goal is to explore the transition in terms of type, context and impact. At this stage, the counsellor attempts to develop a facilitative relationship by using appropriate attending, listening (especially empathy), responding and focusing skills. In the second or Understanding phase, the counsellor tries to facilitate understanding of the issues underlying the transition by having the client examine him or herself including coping resources, his or her environment and the characteristics of the transition. Counsellor skills are intended to promote clarification of the issues for the client and include interpretation, identification of themes, confrontation and presentation of information (e.g., information about transitions) as appropriate. The goal of the third and final stage is to help the client cope more effectively with the transition by taking appropriate action (or inaction). The three major sets of variables which are posited to intermediate between the transition and its resolution (i.e., those which characterize the transition, the individual and his or her environment) need to be assessed in terms of assets/resources and liabilities and interventions designed accordingly. Among the strategies which the counsellor may use to influence the client are problem solving, teaching coping skills, structuring support and individual or group counselling.

Conceptually, Schlossberg (1984) divides the transition process itself into three major phases: "the introduction, during which time the individual is pervaded by the transition; a middle period of disruption, in which the individual is a bit at sea as old norms and relationships are changing and new ones are in process; and a final period in which the individual integrates the transition" (p.61). Within her helping model, the three stages of the counselling process would seem to correspond with the three phases of the transition process. In other words, during the introductory phase of the transition which is marked by pervasiveness, the most appropriate interventions for the counsellor to make would rely on the skills of the first or Exploration stage of the counselling process. Similarly, the skills to promote coping would be used during the final or integration phase of the transition. However, it should be noted that movement through the transition phases toward final constructive integration is not automatic and it is by examining the resources and deficits in each particular case that the counsellor, together with the client, can decide what interventions would best facilitate the process of assimilation.

Similarly, others have attempted to match interventions with the point at which the client appears to be in the process of assimilating the transition. According to Brammer (1991), in the early phases of a transition when an individual is experiencing shock and temporary immobilization, it is extremely important to assess the nature and severity of the transition event accurately, assess the person's coping resources, decide on the best form of help needed and act in a directly helpful way so as to promote stabilization and resolution of the emotional impact of the event. It is especially important to provide support by listening attentively and empathically and by allowing the individual to express his or her feelings. At the second critical point which is marked by cyclical feelings including sadness, relief, elation and despair and by use of psychological defenses such as denial, fantasy and rationalization, it is not only important to continue providing support through active listening and encouraging expression of emotions, but it is also helpful to have the individual describe body experiences, such as pains and pleasures, and to provide reassurance that the contradictory feelings the person is experiencing are normal in certain kinds of loss as well. At critical point three which is characterized by efforts to minimize feelings through denial, disbelief and rationalization, the person begins to lose confidence and slowly becomes depressed. It is important again to acknowledge that this is a normal reaction to loss, a reactive depression, and that moderately sad feelings are to be expected. In addition, the counsellor needs to listen empathically to his or her feelings of fear, anger, guilt and frustration and to help the person maintain his or her self-esteem as well as manage his or her increasingly depressive moods (e.g., through maintaining normal health routines). At the fourth critical point, the individual is usually mildly to moderately depressed. It is useful to encourage the individual to go with his or her moods, to nourish the self, to keep a journal, to spend time alone as well as with supportive others so that the individual may eventually let go of the past and take on new attitudes and behaviours. Cognitive restructuring could appropriately be used at this stage. If the depression becomes chronic or more severe during this stage, consideration should be given to referral to a professional such as a psychiatrist as a combination of psychological methods and medication may be in order. At critical point five, the individual begins to talk of taking hold of tasks and making new plans although these are tentative. The person seems more optimistic and generally happier, though still fragile. However, it is important to note that as the individual moves out of his or her lethargy and has more energy, there is a greater likelihood that the person will entertain suicidal thoughts and actions and the counsellor should be alert for signs of possible self-destruction. So when the client starts to talk of making changes, the counsellor should encourage these behaviours by helping him or her set goals and make realistic plans. At the same time, it is important to recognize any tendencies toward relapse, accepting them and helping the client deal with them. The sixth stage is critical because it is at this point that the growth process that was begun earlier continues or dies. At this point, the counsellor needs to reinforce the positive renewal process, help the client to state goals positively and precisely and encourage him or her to reflect back on what was learned that can be used to deal with similar changes more effectively in the future.

Livneh (1986b), in proposing a number of interventions to be used in assisting a person with a disability as he or she progresses through the stages suggested by his model, recommends that the counsellor be flexible in his or her orientation. "The choice of specific approaches and methods depends on the client's needs; the degree of observed or inferred psychosocial impact; the onset, nature and progression of the disability; the client's support system; the practitioner's acquaintance and mastery of different intervention methods and techniques, and so on" (p. 6). He also suggests that in order to be helpful, the counsellor must have come to terms with his or her own reactions to loss, grief and disability and that he or she must be able to recognize the stage(s) in which the client is operating. Finally, as a rule of thumb, he suggests that the more affective and/or insightful counselling interventions (e.g., as in client-centred counselling, Gestalt therapy) seem to be more helpful in the early stages of the assimilation process while the more cognitive-behavioural and action oriented approaches (e.g., as in behavioural therapy, reality therapy) seem to be appropriate for the later stages. This seems to be consistent with Schlossberg's (1984) framework for helping people in transition.

When working with an individual who has recently acquired a disability and is experiencing shock and anxiety following the trauma, Livneh (1986b) suggests that it is important to listen empathically, provide support and reassurance, offer a careful explanation of the ongoing treatment procedures, allow the client to ventilate feelings and perform muscle relaxation procedures and breathing exercises when anxiety seems to be overwhelming. When defenses become mobilized and denial and bargaining are used as a means of self-protection, Livneh (1986b) suggests that a variety of intervention strategies should be entertained, from initially complying with a client's denial attempts by adopting a neutral attitude, neither encouraging denial nor arguing with the client, to confronting him or her more directly. The counsellor should provide relevant information about the client's impairment as appropriate, taking care not to destroy hopes of recovery or improvement. Gradually, the client should be gently confronted by pointing out inconsistencies and discrepancies in overt behaviours, verbal and nonverbal behaviours, etc. (e.g., through use of Gestalt therapy techniques). The counsellor may encourage the client to fantasize about future activities and tasks and reinforce behaviour which is incompatible with denial. Livneh suggests that when the client is faced with the emotional pain accompanying the initial realization or recognition of his or her loss, the counsellor should encourage expression and clarification of any feelings of depression, guilt or shame while listening in a nonjudgmental way. In addition, one or more of the following approaches may be used as appropriate. The counsellor may help the client develop an awareness of his or her strengths and resources and reinforce positive self-statements and constructive efforts. Tendencies to withdraw or to be dependent should be discouraged. The counsellor may reinforce interpersonal and social skill acquisition and behaviours by the withdrawn client. Stress management and relaxation training can be used when acute grief reactions are observed. Short-term, concrete, and limited goals should be set and rational-emotive therapy techniques may be used to

interrupt the client's irrational beliefs, as manifested i
her verbalizations and associated feelings of hopelessn_ and
despair. For the client who manifests internalized anger
reactions, Livneh (1986b) suggests that the client should be
encouraged and even taught to verbalize, ventilate and release
pent-up anger in a socially-sanctioned manner. Role-playing
may be used to enact anger-causing situations. When the client
begins to show signs of retaliation or rebellion by using both
direct and indirect methods of externalizing anger and
aggressiveness, Livneh (1986b) suggests that the counsellor
should try to understand the origin of these asocial behaviours
and change them through some of the methods to deal with
anger described above as well as by refraining from moralizing
and initially avoiding any direct confrontation, teaching the
client to channel his or her anger into productive and useful
activities, teaching the client to take responsibility for his or her
actions, teaching relaxation techniques to diffuse the anger and
contracting with the client to decrease his or her angry
behaviours. For the client with a disability who reaches the final
phase involving reintegration, Livneh (1986b) suggests that the
counsellor might use a number of physical, psychological, social,
vocational and avocational strategies. Along with encouraging
acceptance of the finality and permanency of the physical
disability and the loss of the old self, the counsellor might help
the client work toward realization of his or her actual functional
limitations and existing strengths. In addition, the counsellor
might help the client to clarify his or her values regarding the
functional limitations imposed by the disability, possibly
replacing them with new ones. The client should be encouraged
to develop a sense of personal responsibility and internal control
of his or her life. Concrete and time-limited goals should be set
followed by rehearsal of possible outcomes. The use of humour
should be encouraged and problem solving and decision-making
skills should be taught where necessary. New and appropriate
behaviours should be discussed and modelled, possibly by
encouraging the client to participate in a group for individuals
with similar disabilities or in family counselling. Finally, the
client should be helped to change and restructure the
environment (i.e., at home, work, recreation) to suit his or her
needs, particularly with regard to mobility or sensory
impairments. The client should be helped to explore further

and solve real problems, particularly by setting realistic goals and priorities in the personal, social and vocational domains and by implementing strategies to reach those goals.

Although it might appear that by being familiar with the phases of assimilation, the counsellor might intervene at each stage relatively easily by mechanically linking an intervention to a phase, it is important to recognize the need to maintain a flexible approach to intervention. As noted earlier, individuals frequently relapse, become stuck or never work through the transition process to a favourable outcome. As Brammer and Abrego (1981) and Schlossberg (1981, 1984) point out, various factors mediate between the transition event and the eventual outcome and it is only by continually assessing the client's perceptions as well as his or her assets and liabilities at any particular point in time that the counsellor can decide on the most appropriate action to take.

The models for counselling during periods of transition described previously (i.e., Brammer, 1991; Livneh, 1986b; Schlossberg, 1984) vary in the degree to which they emphasize social support as an aspect of intervention. Furthermore, social support is generally neglected in traditional approaches to counselling although it has been shown to have a significant impact on the individual's ability to cope with stress. Consequently, without intending to diminish the importance of helping clients in transition acquire other coping skills (e.g., for restructuring cognitions, reducing physiological distress or solving problems), interventions to build social support are specifically highlighted in this section.

Brammer (1991) describes five steps in the process of helping a client build social support:

1. Conduct an inventory of the supportive people in the network;
2. Assess the various types of support available and the current levels of satisfaction with them;
3. Identify and rate on a scale of 1-5 the support functions of each support person;
4. Decide on changes to be made in the network;
5. Help the client acquire skills to make the desired changes in his or her network.

In conducting an assessment of social support, efforts can be made to gather information in a number of areas including the structure of the social support network (e.g., size, interconnectedness, density, and accessibility), the nature or content of the support provided, the provider of the support (i.e., family member, friend, professional, stranger), the subjective appraisal of the perceived support, the length of time the support has been available, the activities involved in the provision of support and the process by which the individual develops, nurtures, and uses supportive ties. No single instrument is available to provide such an appraisal. However, some informal and some formal procedures may be used to obtain a more comprehensive assessment of the network and the social support provided. Some informal assessment approaches are outlined here while more formal assessment procedures are described elsewhere (e.g., see Morosan and Pearson, 1981; Robertson, 1987, 1988). It should be noted that not all procedures will be appropriate for all clients. In the case of the person with a disability, the procedure selected will depend on the disability and where possible, adaptations in conducting the assessment should be made.

The simplest method of gaining information about a client's psychosocial assets is to ask relevant questions in the course of the counselling interview. Clients should be asked about their families and friends, the nature of each relationship, its potential for supportive or conflicting behaviours and the perceived adequacy of these relationships. Some researchers (Brown, Bhrolchain and Harris, 1975) found that simply having a number of confidants is highly predictive of client satisfaction with the network. It is important to keep in mind that a lack of close ties or a confidant is usually a significant indicator of some form of difficulty because of the potential impact of the social network in aiding or abetting client progress. In the case of disability, the client might be asked about the network's interpretations of his or her disability, their expectations for treatment, and their reactions to the goals, plans and methods set up during the course of counselling (Gottlieb, 1983). The counsellor can then periodically assess the primary network's response to counselling interventions.

A number of other methods might be used to validate or supplement the information gained from the interview. One of these involves the use of a journal. Here, the client is given specific instructions about what is to be recorded in the journal (e.g., the name of any person with whom he or she has a conversation, the topic discussed, feelings about the encounter and/or the person, the name of any person who helped to complete specific tasks, and what the person did to help). The journal should be completed daily and later examined to identify various aspects of the support system.

Several structured activities (Ashinger, 1985; Gottlieb, 1983, 1984) have been developed to guide people through the process of identifying their social resources, exploring their perceptions of the types and quality of the support they give and receive and planning changes that might strengthen the supportive aspects of their lives. Gottlieb (1984) asks clients to map their primary social networks along certain structural dimensions including size, composition, degree of correctedness (density), and geographic dispersion, and along specific process dimensions including types of helping exchanges, degree of reciprocity in these exchanges, and levels of relational intimacy. Following this, clients are asked to assess the types (socializing and companionship, emotional support, advice and guidance, tangible aid, and esteem support) and extent of support they exchange with their network members. By first examining the map for structural characteristics (e.g., size, density, and intimacy of relationships) and later examining access to the five types of support, the client and counsellor can then focus on planning changes in the structure and supportive processes of the client's network. Eventually, the client may be asked to specify two network/support objectives, and the client and counsellor together may develop a list of practical steps that could be taken to achieve these changes. Logs or diaries as outlined previously may be used to chart the effects of these changes on a daily or weekly basis.

Depending on the nature of the client's support network and the kinds of changes desired, intervention strategies may be aimed at various levels of the support system (Pearson, 1983; Robertson, 1987,1988):

1. Efforts may be directed to improving the client's interpersonal awareness and/or skills as a lack of these may be hindering his or her success in forming and maintaining supportive relationships. Focus on this level takes

precedence when adequate informal support resources actually or potentially exist but the client for some reason is unable to access or maintain them;

2. Efforts may be aimed at increasing the responsiveness and/or resources of the client's existing support persons through direct intervention (e.g., by raising their awareness of the client's need for support or by teaching them how to provide appropriate support). Focus on the client's existing support resources takes precedence when improvements or additions to support resources already available to the client are needed;

3. Efforts may be made to link a client with a surrogate, in contrast to a natural, support system (e.g., mutual help groups, self-help groups). Focus on developing links with surrogate support systems are preferable when the natural support system is unable or unwilling to provide needed support for the client. In this case, the client is encouraged to change the structure and quality of the network by building new relationships.

SUMMARY AND RECOMMENDATIONS

In this chapter, a general framework for understanding psychosocial issues associated with various types of life transitions is presented on the assumption that such a framework is likely to be helpful in counselling individuals with physical disabilities. Although specific emphasis is placed on the transition to physical illness or disability, it is argued that the framework could be useful in counselling persons with physical disabilities who are undergoing other types of life transitions. The transition process itself is examined in terms of various phases of assimilation. The influence of cognitive appraisals in mediating individual responses to the transition event is considered. Other factors affecting the outcome of the transition process including those pertaining to the transition, the environment, and the individual are outlined. More specifically, characteristics of the transition which affect outcome include the type of transition (anticipated, unanticipated, chronic hassle, nonevent), the context in which it occurs, the impact, the trigger (precipitator), the timing (on-time or off-time), the source

)r external), role change (gain or loss), duration t, temporary, or uncertain), previous experience with a similar transition and concurrent stress. Both the physical and psychosocial environment play an influential role in shaping responses to a transition event. Some characteristics of the individual in transition which affect outcome include age and stage of life, state of health, personality, cultural background, commitments and values and coping responses. A framework such as this lends itself to the development of interventions for counselling individuals in transition and specifically those adapting to physical disability.

A number of recommendations for counselling people with physical disabilities can be made on the basis of the work presented here:

1. Rehabilitation counsellors should become knowledgable about transition processes, the adaptive tasks demanded by various types of life transition and factors which mediate between the transition event and outcome;
2. Rehabilitation counsellors need to be sensitive to the various life transitions facing individuals with physical disabilities in addition to the transition to the disability itself. They need to recognize the influence of the physical disability on adaptation to other transitions as well as the influence of other transition events on adaptation to the disability itself. This interactive process goes on across the life span;
3. Rehabilitation counsellors need to be able to assess how the client is coping with the transition process at any particular point in time and design appropriate interventions accordingly;
4. An assessment of the client's social support system should form a part of the overall assessment of the client and the resulting information should be used in designing intervention plans. Changes in social support should be monitored on an on-going basis;
5. Interventions should be directed to various parts of the client's psychosocial world in order to affirm, use, and strengthen the social support given and received by clients as necessary;
6. Clients should be helped to overcome their own barriers to

accessing available support;
7. Network members' attitudes and behavioural responses to thecounselling process itself should be monitored and members should be offered various forms of support as required. Where necessary, members should be taught how to be more supportive to one another;
8. Counsellors and rehabilitation practitioners should develop psycho-educational programmes to help clients and/or their families acquire needed coping skills;
9. Counsellors and rehabilitation practitioners should actively promote the provision of surrogate sources of support such as peer-help and mutual-aid groups to clients with common disabilities;
10. Although various studies have been conducted on the process of adaptation to a number of physical disabilities, research is needed on the process of assimilating other types of life transitions by those with physical disabilities.

REFERENCES

Abramson, L., Seligman, M. and Teasdale, J. (1978) 'Learned Helplessness in Humans: Critique and Reformulation', *Journal of Abnormal Psychology, 87,* 165-180.

Ahrons, C.R. (1980) 'Divorce: A Crisis of Family Transition and Changes', *Family Relations, 29,* 533-540.

Ashinger, P. (1985) 'Using Social Networks in Counselling', *Journal of Counseling and Development, 63,* 519-521.

Borgen, W.A., Amundson, N.E. and Biela, P.M. (1987) 'The Experience of Unemployment of the Physically Disabled', in R.I. Brown (ed), *Natcon 14: Vocational Counselling in Rehabilitation (Part I),* Minister of Supply and Services Canada, Ottawa, ON.

Brammer, L. (1991) *How to Cope with Life Transitions: The Challenge of Personal Change,* Hemisphere, Washington, DC.

Brammer, L. and Abrego, P. (1981) 'Intervention Strategies for Coping with Transitions', *The Counseling Psychologist, 9,* 19-35.

Brammer, L.M. and Shostrom, E.L. (1977) *Therapeutic Psychology: Fundamentals of Counseling and Psychotherapy* (3rd ed.), Prentice-Hall, Englewood Cliffs, NJ.

Brown, G., Bhrolchain, M. and Harris, T. (1975) 'Social Class and Psychiatric Disturbance Among Women in an Urban Population', *Sociology, 9,* 225-254.

Cohen, F. and Lazarus, R.S. (1979) 'Coping with the Stresses of

Illness', in G.C. Stone, F. Cohen and N.E. Adler (eds), *Health Psychology - A Handbook*, Jossey-Bass, San Francisco.

Coyne, J.C., Wortman, C.B. and Lehman, D.R. (1988) 'The Other Side of Support: Emotional Overinvolvement and Miscarried Helping', in B. H. Gottlieb (ed), *Marshalling Social Support*, Sage, Newbury Park, CA.

Davidson, T.N., Bowden, L. and Tholen, D. (1979) 'Social Support as a Moderator of Burn Rehabilitation', *Archives of Physical Medicine and Rehabilitation*, 60, 556.

Davis, S.E., Anderson, T., Linkowski, D.C., Berger, K. and Feinstein, C F. (1985) 'Developmental Tasks and Transitions of Adolescents with Chronic Illnesses and Disabilities', *Rehabilitation Counseling Bulletin*, 29, 69-80.

Di Matteo, R. and Hays, R. (1981) 'Social Support and Serious Illness', in B.H. Gottlieb (ed), *Social Networks and Social Support*, Sage, Beverly Hills, CA.

Dimond, M. (1979) 'Social Support and Adaptation to Chronic Illness: The Case of Maintenance Hemodialysis', *Research in Nursing and Health*, 2, 101-108.

Doehrman, S.R. (1977) 'Psycho-social Aspects of Recovery from Coronary Heart Disease: A Review', *Social Science and Medicine*, 11, 199-218.

Dushensko, T.W. (1981) 'Cystic Fibrosis: A Medical Review and Critique of the Psychological Literature', *Social Science and Medicine*, 15E, 43-56.

Egan, G. (1975) *The Skilled Helper* (1st ed.), Brooks/Cole, Monterey, CA.

Egan, G. (1986) *The Skilled Helper* (3rd ed.), Brooks/Cole, Pacific Grove, CA.

Erikson, E. (1963) *Childhood and Society* (2nd ed.), Norton, New York.

Fengler, A.P. and Goodrich, N. (1979) 'Wives of Elderly Disabled Men: Hidden Patient', *Gerontologist*, 19, 175-183.

Finlayson, A. (1976) 'Social Support Networks as Coping Resources: Lay Help and Consultation Patterns Used by Women in Husband's Post-infarction Careers', *Social Science and Medicine*, 10, 97-103.

Gottlieb, B.H. (1983) *Social Support Strategies: Guidelines for Mental Health Practice*, Sage Publications, Beverly Hills, CA.

Gottlieb, B.H. (1984) 'Assessing and Strengthening the Preventive Impact of Social Support', Unpublished Manuscript, The University of Guelph, Guelph, Ontario.

Heath, R.W. and Levin, P. (1991). 'Cultural Sensitivity in the Design and Evaluation of Early Intervention Programmes', in D. Mitchell and R.I. Brown (eds), *Early Intervention Studies for Young Children with Special Needs*, Chapman and Hall, London.

Hopson, B. (1981) 'Response to Papers by Schlossberg, Brammer, and Abrego', *The Counseling Psychologist*, 9, 36-40.

Hopson, B. and Adams, J. (1976) 'Towards an Understanding of Transition: Defining Some Boundaries of Transition Dynamics', in J. Adams, J. Hayes and B. Hopson (eds), *Transitions: Understanding and Managing Personal Change*, Martin Robertson, London.

Hopson, B. and Adams, J. (1977) 'Transitions: Defining Some Boundaries', in J. Adams, J. Hayes and B. Hopson (eds), *Transition*, Allenheld and Osman, Montclair, NJ.

Hymovich, D. and Baker, C.D. (1985) 'The Needs, Concerns, and Coping of Parents of Children with Cystic Fibrosis', *Family Relations*, 34, 91-98.

Ingram, M.A. (1989) 'Psycho-social Aspects of Breast Cancer', *Journal of Applied Rehabilitation Counseling*, 20, 23-27.

Kaplan, R.M. and Toshima, M.T. (1990) 'The Functional Effects of Social Relationships on Chronic Illnesses and Disability', in B.R. Sarason, I.G. Sarason and G.R. Pierce (eds), *Social Support: An Interactional View*, John Wiley and Sons, New York, NY.

Kivnick, H.Q. (1985) 'Disability and Psychosocial Development in Old Age', *Rehabilitation Counseling Bulletin*, 29, 123-134.

Kubler-Ross, E. (1975) *Death: The Final Stage of Growth*, Prentice-Hall, Englewood Cliffs, NJ.

Lazarus, R.S. and Folkman, S. (1984) *Stress, Appraisal, and Coping*, Springer, New York, NY.

Lazarus, R.S. and Launier, R. (1978) 'Stress-related Transactions Between Person and Environment', in L.A. Pervin and M. Lewis (eds), *Perspectives in Interactional Psychology*, Plenum, New York, NY.

Lieberman, M. (1975) 'Adaptive Processes in Late Life', in N. Datan and L. Ginsberg (eds), *Life Span Development Psychology; Normative Life Crises*, Academic Press, New York.

Lindemann, E. (1979) *Beyond Grief: Studies in Crisis Intervention*, Jason Aronson, New York.

Livneh, H. (1986a) 'A Unified Approach to Existing Models of Adaptation to Disability: Part I - A Model of Adaptation', *Journal of Applied Rehabilitation Counseling*, 17, 5-16.

Livneh, H. (1986b) 'A Unified Approach to Existing Models of Adaptation to Disability: Part II - Intervention Strategies', *Journal of Applied Rehabilitation Counseling, 17,* 6-10.

Loveys, B. (1990) 'Transitions in Chronic Illness: The At-risk Role', *Holistic Nursing Practice, 4,* 56-64.

Malmquist, A. and Hagberg, B. (1974) 'Prospective Study of Patients in Chronic-hemodialysis. 5. Follow Up Study of 13 Patients in Home-dialysis', *Journal of Psychosomatic Medicine, 8,* 495-519.

Maruta, T., Osbourne, D., Swanson, D.W. and Hallnig, J.M. (1981) 'Chronic Pain Patients and Spouses - Marital and Sexual Adjustment', *Mayo Clinic Proceedings, 56,* 307-310.

Moos, R.H. and Schaefer, J.A. (1984) 'The Crisis of Physical Illness: An Overview and Conceptual Approach', in R.H. Moos (ed), *Coping with Physical Illness 2: New Perspectives,* Plenum Medical Book Co., London.

Moos, R.H. and Tsu, V. (1976) 'Human Competence and Coping: An Overview', in R.H. Moos (ed), *Human Adaptation: Coping with Life Crises,* Heath, Lexington, MA.

Morosan, E. and Pearson, R. (1981) 'Upon Whom Do You Depend: Mapping Personal Support Systems', *Canada's Mental Health,* 1-4.

Myers, J.E. (1985) 'Using Links to Help Older Disabled Persons with Transitions', *Rehabilitation Counseling Bulletin, 29,* 143-149.

Parkes, V. and Weiss, R. (1983) *Recovery from Bereavement,* Basic Books, New York.

Patterson, J. (1985) 'Critical Factors Affecting Family Compliance with Home Treatment for Children with Cystic Fibrosis', *Family Relations, 34,* 79-90.

Pearlin, L.I. (1980) Life Strains and Psychological Distress Among Adults , in N.J. Smelser and E.H. Erikson (eds), *Themes of Work and Love in Adulthood* (pp. 174 - 192), Howard University Press, Cambridge, MA.

Pearlin, L.I. and Aneshensel, C.S. (1986) 'Coping and Social Supports: Their Functions and Applications', in L. Aiken and D. Mechanic (eds), *Applications of Social Science to Clinical Medicine and Health Policy* (pp. 417-437), Rutgers University Press, New Brunswick, NJ.

Pearlin, L. and Schooler, C. (1978) 'The Structure of Coping', *Journal of Health and Social Behavior, 19,* 2-21.

Pearson, R.E. (1983) 'Support Groups: A Conceptualization', *The Personnel and Guidance Journal, 61(6),* 361-364.

Porritt, D. (1979) 'Social Support in Crisis: Quantity or Quality?', *Social Science and Medicine, 13A,* 715-721.

Power, P.W., Hershenson, D.B. and Schlossberg, N.K. (1985) 'Midlife

Transition and Disability', *Rehabilitation Counseling Bulletin*, 29, 100-111.

Robertson, S.E. (1987) 'Social Support and its Implications for Counselling Disabled People', in R.I. Brown (ed), *Natcon 14: Vocational Counselling in Rehabilitation (Part I)*, Minister of Supply and Services Canada, Ottawa, ON.

Robertson, S.E. (1988) 'Social Support: Implications for Counselling', *International Journal for the Advancement of Counselling*, 11, 313-321.

Saulnier, K. (1982) 'Networks, Change and Crisis: The Web of Support', *Canadian Journal of Community Psychology*, 1, 5-23.

Schlossberg, N.K. (1981) 'A Model for Analyzing Human Adaptation to Transition', *The Counseling Psychologist*, 9 (2), 2-18.

Schlossberg, N.K. (1984) *Counseling Adults in Transition*, Springer Publishing, New York.

Schweitzer, N.J. (1982) 'Coping with Stigma: An Integrated Approach to Counseling Physically Disabled Persons', *Rehabilitation Counseling Bulletin*, 25(4), 204-211.

Seligman, M. (1975) *Helplessness: On Depression, Development, and Death*, W.H. Freeman, San Francisco.

Simonton, O.C. and Simonton, S. (1975) 'Belief Systems and Management of Emotional Aspects of Maligning', *Journal of Transpersonal Psychology*, 7, 29-47.

Smith, E. (1985) 'Ethnic Minorities: Life Stress, Social Support, and Mental Health Issues', *The Counseling Psychologist*, 13, 537-579.

Vargo, J.W. (1979) 'The Disabled Wife and Mother: Suggested Goals for Family Counselling', *Canadian Counsellor*, 13, 108-111.

Vargo, J.W. (1989) "In the House of my Friend': Dealing with Disability', *International Journal for the Advancement of Counseling*, 12, 281-287.

Ware, L.A. and Carper, M. (1982) 'Living with Alzheimer's Disease Patients: Family Stress and Coping Mechanisms', *Psychotherapy: Theory, Research, and Practice*, 19, 472-481.

Watzlawick, P. and Coyne, J.C. (1980) 'Depression Following Stroke: Brief Problem-Focussed Family Treatment', *Family Process*, 19, 13-18.

Wesolowski, M.D. (1987) 'Differences in Sizes of Social Networks of Rehabilitation Clients Versus Those of Nonclients', *Rehabilitation Counseling Bulletin*, 32, 17-27.

Chapter Seven

COUNSELLING FAMILY MEMBERS OF PEOPLE WITH DISABILITIES

Garry Hornby

INTRODUCTION

> Handicap is beyond doubt a disruptive event in the life of the family as a whole and it therefore has repercussions for the lives of each family member (Kew, 1975, p. 156).

Professionals who work with people with disabilities need to bear in mind that the vast majority of their clients are members of families, which, in most cases, are their main source of long-term support. It is now widely accepted that families both affect and are affected by their members who have disabilities in various ways (Sameroff and Chandler, 1975). However, many practitioners consider themselves to be working with individual clients quite independently from their families. They consider that their work will only affect clients themselves. However, since the application of family systems theory to families with handicapped members (Coopersmith, 1984) this view is more difficult to justify. Some writers go so far as to suggest that an intervention with any family member is in fact an intervention with the whole family (Berger and Foster, 1986). Others go even further and claim that treatment of individuals, without regard to family functioning, may result in an increase in the problems experienced by the family as a whole (Chilman, Nunnally and Cox, 1988).

This chapter will discuss the impact that a person with a disability can have on other family members, such as mothers, fathers, siblings and grandparents, and describe various approaches to preventing or ameliorating any negative effects which may result. This will include discussion of:

1. Models of family functioning;
2. The process of adaptation to the disability;
3. Effects on members of the family;
4. The major needs of family members;
5. Individual, group and family interventions, and the skills, attitudes and knowledge needed by professionals in order to work effectively with families of people with disabilities.

MODELS OF FAMILY FUNCTIONING

Several different models have emerged in recent years in the social sciences which have begun to have an impact on research and practice with families of people with disabilities. Three of these are described below. These are:

1. The transactional model;
2. The ecological model, and;
3. Family systems theory.

Transactional Model

In this model, development is believed to result from a continual interplay between a changing organism and a changing environment (Sameroff and Chandler, 1975). Thus, families are considered to both affect and be affected by their member who has a handicap. Also, as people with disabilities pass through different developmental stages they will affect their families in different ways. For example, an infant with a disability will have a different effect on parents than an adolescent. Likewise, the effect parents have on their child with special needs will depend on the particular stage in the life cycle in which they find themselves. That is, a child with a handicapping condition, who is the first born child of young, recently married parents is in a very different situation to a child with the same condition born to older parents who already have several other children.

Ecological Model

In this model, human development and behaviour cannot be understood independently of the context in which it occurs. Environment influences behaviour and this occurs at several levels (Bronfenbrenner, 1979). Thus, the effects on parents of caring for a child with special needs are strongly influenced by the environment in which they are living, including the extended family, services available and community attitudes. The family of a child with a handicap is considered to constitute a microsystem with the child, parents and sibling reciprocally influencing each other. This family microsystem is influenced by the mesosystem in which it is embedded. The mesosystem comprises the range of settings in which the family actively participates, such as the extended family, school and work settings. The mesosystem is itself influenced by the exosystem. The exosystem level consists of settings in which the family is not actively involved but in which events occur that affect the family, such as the mass media, education system and voluntary agencies. Finally, there is the macrosystem which comprises the ideological systems inherent in the social institutions of a particular society such as religious, economic and political beliefs (Mitchell, 1985). Thus, the development and behaviour of a family with a person who has a disability is influenced not only by interactions within its own microsystem but also by its interactions with other levels of the entire social system.

Family Systems Theory

In this model, the behaviour of family members is considered to be a function of the system of which they are a part. A change in the family system will inevitably lead to a change in the behaviour of each of the family members. Likewise, a change in an individual's behaviour will cause the family system to change. However, the functioning of the family system is considered to comprise more than just a summation of the contributions of its individual members. Intervention at the level of the family system is therefore likely to have more impact than intervention aimed at one of its members (Berger,

1984). The implication of this for professionals is that the whole family system needs to be considered when instituting a treatment programme.

In order to elucidate the various elements of the family system, a Family Systems Conceptual Framework has been developed by Turnbull and her associates (Turnbull, Summers, and Brotherson, 1984; Turnbull and Turnbull, 1986). This framework is made up of four components. First, there is the family interaction component which refers to the relationships that occur among and between the various sub-systems of family members. That is, the spousal sub-system (husband-wife interactions), the parental sub-system (parent-child interactions), and the sibling sub-system (child-child interactions). It also refers to extra-familial interactions such as those between children and grandparents or those between a father and his workmates. Then, there is the family resources component which consists of descriptive elements of the family, including characteristics of the disability such as type and severity; characteristics of the family such as size, cultural background and socio-economic status; and personal characteristics such as health and coping styles. The family functions component refers to the different types of needs which the family provides, such as economic, physical care, recuperation, socialization, affection, self-definition, educational and vocational needs. Finally, the family life cycle component represents the sequence of developmental changes that affect families as they progress through various stages in the life cycle, such as unattached adulthood, marriage, birth of children, school-entry, adolescent children, children leaving home, and retirement.

Family life cycle changes affect family functions and resources which in turn affect family interaction patterns. That is, the four components of the family system are interdependent. This suggests that an understanding of all four components of the family system is needed when considering the impact of an intervention on the family. The family systems conceptual framework can therefore be used to provide a thorough analysis of families with members who have disabilities before an intervention is begun.

ADAPTATION PROCESS

Several models have been proposed to explain the process which people experience in adapting to a family member with a disability (see for example: Seligman, 1979; Wright, Granger and Sameroff, 1984). Most writers describe a stage model of adaptation to loss similar to the one proposed by Hornby (1982) which is outlined below. Feedback on this model, from a large number of parents and professionals, has confirmed its value in elucidating the process. Although there is some debate among professionals as to the accuracy of such a stage model (Blacher, 1984), it has been this writer's experience that many parents gain considerable comfort from being made aware of such a conceptualization of the adaptation process.

In this model, it is suggested that the process of adaptation can be viewed as a continuum of reactions, beginning at the diagnosis, through which people pass in order to come to terms with the disabling condition. The various reactions will now be described in the order in which they may be experienced.

1. Shock: People report feeling confusion, numbness, disorganization and helplessness. They often say that they were unable to take in much of what they were told at this time. This state typically lasts from a few hours to a few days.

2. Denial: Disbelief or denial of the reality of the situation often follows the shock reaction. As a temporary coping strategy this is quite healthy. However, prolonged denial can lead to shopping around for a more favourable diagnosis which, if found, could retard the adaptation process.

3. Anger: People may search for a cause of the disability. They may blame themselves or hospital staff and experience anger which may be displaced onto a spouse, a child, or onto professionals involved. Underlying the anger may be feelings of guilt about somehow being responsible for the disability.

4. Sadness: People may feel depressed, despairing, or just very sad. This is a reaction which is often reported to pervade the whole process to some extent.

5. Detachment: Many people experience a time when they feel empty or flat. Nothing seems to matter. They accept the reality of the disability but have lost some of the meaning of life.

6. Reorganization: This phase is characterized by realism and hope. People consider their "cup is half-full, rather than half-empty".

7. Adaptation: When people have come to terms with the situation they exhibit a mature emotional acceptance of the family member with the disability. They are fully aware of the person's special needs and strive to provide for these. However, he or she is treated, as much as possible, as just another member of the family, which does not revolve around him or her. People may always experience some sadness that a member of their family has a disability but they don't let this interfere with their efforts to make the best out of life.

The adaptation process is considered to be a normal healthy reaction to the diagnosis of disability. People may need only a few days or take many years in which to work through it. It can be viewed as a form of grieving similar to that which follows any traumatic loss.

Many people have said that they experienced feelings associated with more than one phase at certain times. Some do not experience a particular phase, while others report being fixated at one phase for a considerable time before being able to move on. Some people say that they experienced the phases in a different order. Thus, the process is qualitatively different for each person and therefore this model should be viewed only as a general guide and not as a prescription which everybody is expected to follow.

Even after working through the continuum of reactions and having come to terms with the disability, people are likely to experience sadness or grief which may always be present to some extent. This has led some writers to suggest that, rather than a grieving process which can be worked through with feelings to some extent resolved, parents of children with disabilities experience "chronic sorrow" (Olshansky, 1962; Wikler, Wasow and Hatfield, 1981). It is suggested that the various reactions which are evoked such as anger, sadness and denial are not resolved but become an integral part of the parents' emotional life (Max, 1985). Thus, there will be various occasions when these reactions may be re-experienced. This reworking of parental reactions can occur at various transition points in the development of the child with the handicap such as school entry, the onset of puberty, leaving school and leaving home (Wikler, 1981 and 1986). It can also occur when an additional disability is diagnosed at some time later than the original diagnosis (Featherstone, 1981).

An alternative way in which the adaptation process can be viewed, as applied to parents of people with disabilities, has been proposed by Mitchell (1985). Parents are seen as progressing through a series of developmental stages, each of which is characterized by a set of tasks which must be at least partially mastered if they are to successfully adapt to the presence of a person with a handicapping condition in the family. The four broad stages of development proposed are:

1. Initial diagnosis;
2. Infancy and toddlerhood;
3. Childhood and early adolescence
4. Late adolescence and adulthood.

The tasks included in the four stages are listed below.

1. Initial diagnosis:
   a) Deciding whether to pursue aggressive medical care where the infant's life is at risk;
   b) Deciding whether to keep the child or seek alternative care;
   c) Accepting the reality of the handicapping condition;
   d) Coming to terms with one's reactions to disability;
   e) Understanding the nature of the disability, its causation and developmental possibilities;
   f) Maintaining or enhancing self-esteem;
   g) Establishing a positive parenting relationship with the infant;
   h) Coming to terms with the reactions of family, friends and workmates;

i) Maintaining or enhancing relationship with spouse.

2. Infancy and toddlerhood:
   a) Making contact with other families with children with similar disabilities;
   b) Accessing appropriate support services;
   c) Establishing productive working relationships with particular professionals;
   d) Coping with reactions of the broader community;
   e) Becoming familiar with the rights of people with disabilities and their families; acquiring advocacy skills;
   f) Establishing a balanced family and personal life;
   g) Developing competence in facilitating the child's development;
   h) Coping with the day to day tasks of caring for a child with a disability.

3. Childhood and early adolescence:
   a) Participating in decisions regarding special education;
   b) Maintaining working relationships with professionals;
   c) Accepting the prolonged dependence of the child;
   d) Facilitating adaptation of, and to, the community;
   e) Helping the child understand his or her disability.

4. Late adolescence and adulthood:
   a) Accepting the right to independence of the person with the disability;
   b) Accepting the sexuality and need for close relationships outside the family of the person who has the disability;
   c) Accepting that the disabled person may wish to live outside the family home;
   d) Participating in decisions regarding jobs and training;
   e) Becoming familiar with the legal rights of persons with disabilities;
   f) Ensuring satisfactory provision for the person who has the disability when parents are elderly or dead.

The issue is not whether adaptation of family members should be viewed as a continuum of emotional reactions, or characterized by chronic sorrow, or by stages of developmental tasks. Each model focuses attention on, and thus, clarifies, different aspects of the adaptation process. Therefore, they can be considered complementary. Also, each model is useful in providing professionals with some insight into the lives of families with members who have disabilities, thereby helping professionals to develop the understanding necessary for working with them.

EFFECTS ON MEMBERS OF THE FAMILY

The importance of considering the effects on families due to one of their members having a disability has been increasingly realized in recent years. Whereas most of the existing literature refers to effects on parents, the vast majority of research has been conducted with mothers. Comments about fathers, siblings and other family members have typically been gained from surveys conducted with others, whose perceptions of the reactions of other family members may not always be accurate (Byrne, Cunningham and Sloper, 1988). Bearing this reservation in mind the effects on families and their members will now be considered.

Families

The social life of many families with members who have disabilities tends to be restricted (Lonsdale, 1978). Leisure activities such as participation in sports and other clubs and family activities such as visiting friends, having picnics and attending family gatherings are often affected. Many families are restricted in the use they can make of community facilities such as beaches, restaurants and public transport. There are also limitations in the type of holidays which families can take. The extent of the social restriction is greatest when the children are young, when physical handicap or behavioural problems are present and when the degree of handicapping condition is severe (Hornby, 1987). The importance of overnight and day-care for the child with a disability, in allowing families to participate in social activities and thereby recharging their emotional batteries, cannot be over-emphasized.

Families with children who have disabilities have to meet additional expenses (Lonsdale, 1978; Murphy, 1982). These are most often for medical care, clothing and transport. The family's income may be reduced since one parent is prevented from going out to work because of the daily care requirements of the child with the disability. Most countries have various financial benefits available to assist such families. However, surveys have shown that many parents do not receive the benefits to which they are entitled (Hornby, 1987). Professionals must therefore convey to parents, by every means possible, information about the benefits and services for which they are eligible.

Parents

Many parents of children with disabilities are reported to experience marital difficulties (Max, 1985). This is considered to be due to the additional demands of caring for a child with a handicap, though several other related factors may be involved. Spouses may disagree about the child's care or treatment and have insufficient time to resolve their conflicts. Having to deal with various professionals increases the strain, particularly since it is usually the mother who sees the professionals and has to reinterpret the interview for the father. It could be that, because of greater involvement with professionals and the child, mothers sometimes move through the adaptation process more quickly than fathers, creating more room for conflict. Difficulties in sexual relationships may result from a lack of privacy, fatigue, a sense of isolation on the part of each spouse or the fear of producing another child with a handicap (Featherstone, 1981).

Several studies have investigated the prevalence of negative effects on the marital relationship resulting from parenting a child with disabilities. Overall, the results have been inconclusive, with the reports of high marriage breakdown and low marital satisfaction being balanced by findings of average levels of these variables in other studies (Byrne *et al.*, 1988; Furneaux, 1988). One result which has been consistently found is that a stable and satisfying marriage helps to reduce the stress experienced by parents in coping with a child who has a disability (Minnes, 1988). Therefore, it is important that the facilitation of marital relationships is seen as a valid focus for interventions with the family. Also, it is clear that because of the factors discussed above, some parents will need considerable support and counselling at various times if their marriage is to grow and succeed. This assistance may be forthcoming from friends or relations, but if not, professionals should be available to meet the need.

Mothers

Many studies have shown that the bulk of the housework and child care in families with members who have disabilities is carried out by mothers (see Fewell and Vadasy, 1986). Despite the increased demands which a person with a disability makes on these aspects of family life fathers generally do not make a bigger contribution than they make in ordinary families (Byrne *et al.*, 1988; McConachie, 1986). Another fairly consistent and probably related finding is that mothers of children who have disabilities exhibit higher levels of stress than mothers of children who are without handicaps (Minnes, 1988). Some studies have reported that this has led to such mothers suffering a higher incidence of stress-related physical and mental disorders than mothers in ordinary families (Hornby, 1987; Philip and Duckworth, 1982).

Fathers

Fathers generally play a smaller part than mothers in the day-to-day care of their children with disabilities. They also have less contact with professionals since most appointments tend to occur when they are at work. This lower level of interaction with professionals and the child may lead to greater difficulty in coming to terms with the child who has a disability. Fathers may use denial to avoid facing up to the full extent of the handicapping condition or to hide their true feelings about the situation (Featherstone, 1981). Since fathers go off to work during the day and generally have other interests outside the home, their mental health may be less threatened than that of mothers. Thus, fathers are able to have a break away from the situation so that they can return home refreshed, adding emotional stability to the family. However, work and other interests can also provide a haven for fathers, thereby reducing their positive influence on the family.

In the last few years there has been increasing interest in the effects on fathers of having a son or daughter with a disability (Lamb, 1983). Very little research has been conducted specifically with such fathers so reviews of the literature have tended to rely mainly on information from studies of mothers and of mother/father differences. The impression gained from this literature, of the effect on fathers of parenting a child with a disability, is generally a negative one. Fathers are reported to have difficulty in accepting disability, particularly if it occurs in a son or if the child has a severe handicap. Also, fathers are reported to experience a higher level of depression, personality difficulties and marital relationship problems than fathers of children who have no handicaps (Brotherson *et al.*, 1986; Meyer, 1986). However, one review of the literature has concluded that considerably more research needs to be conducted with fathers before any such definitive statements can be made (Bristol and Gallagher, 1986).

Whereas mothers are generally considered to need more breaks from the constant care of the child who has a disability, and more interests outside the home, fathers are thought to need more support in coming to terms with the disability (Lamb, 1983). However, fathers are often reluctant to accept involvement in counselling or support groups. Providing the necessary support to fathers therefore presents a real challenge to professionals. Perhaps a start can be made by scheduling appointments at times convenient for both parents to attend.

Siblings

Most parents of children with disabilities worry about the possible harmful effects on their other children. There are several factors which can contribute to sibling maladjustment (Seligman and Darling, 1989). Siblings, especially females, are often given caretaking responsibility for their handicapped brother or sister who has a disability. If this is excessive, it can lead to siblings assuming parental roles, missing out on some of the developmental stages necessary for normal growth, and experiencing considerable resentment and anger. Children may also wonder whether parents will expect them to care for their sibling who has a disability in later life and may worry about finding a spouse who would be willing to share such a responsibility (Featherstone, 1981). A related concern is that many siblings feel the need to overachieve to compensate for parental disappointment over the child with the disability.

Another factor is the concern over "catching" the disability. Young siblings may fear that they too will develop mental handicap, go blind, or even die as the child with the disability has done. As siblings reach adolescence, some worry about the future possibility of producing children with handicaps themselves. The siblings considered to be most at risk are: those from small families, or girls from large families; those who are younger than the child with the handicap and of the same sex; and those whose brother or sister has either a severe handicap, or whose disability is ambiguous (Crnic and Leconte, 1986; Simeonsson and McHale, 1981).

There are, however, frequent reports of the positive effects on sibling adjustment of having a family member who has a disability. Parents often remark on the tolerance, humility and concern for others displayed by siblings. One example of this is that siblings frequently choose careers in the helping professions such as teaching or social work (Furneaux, 1988).

Communication within the family is important. If parents develop open, honest relationships within the family, then their children's achievements and positive and negative feelings will be acknowledged. If not, anger, guilt, feelings of isolation, or resentment about the time parents spend with the child with the disability may build up and remain unresolved. Parents should limit caregiving responsibilities and schedule special time for siblings. They should make sure that siblings have a good understanding of their brother's or sister's disability and are involved as much as possible in discussions and decisions about him or her (Powell and Ogle, 1985).

Grandparents

A common source of support for the family is the grandparents of the child who has a disability, particularly the maternal grandparents. However, the diagnosis of disability often leads to a breakdown in the relationship between generations (Max, 1985; Sonnek, 1986). This may be due to the difficulties of grandparents in adapting to the handicap themselves. Therefore, it may be helpful to also make supportive counselling available to grandparents and involve them, along with parents, in conferences about the child (Seligman and Darling, 1989).

BASIC NEEDS OF FAMILY MEMBERS

Four basic needs of families of people with disabilities are discussed below. These are:
1. Having the diagnosis of disability, or the results of assessments, communicated to them in a sensitive and constructive manner;
2. Obtaining information about the handicapping condition, the services available;
3. Facilitating the development of the person with the disability;
4. Receiving emotional support and help in understanding feelings and reactions;
5. Meeting other members of exceptional families who are in a similar position to themselves.

Receiving the results of diagnoses or assessments

The vast majority of people prefer to be told diagnostic or assessment results by a professional who communicates empathy, sensitivity, openness, and a positive yet realistic outlook. This person should be knowledgeable about the possible causes and likely consequences of the disability and of the services available. People prefer to be told as soon as possible after a diagnosis is made, or a problem becomes apparent, with both parents together and, if appropriate, with the family member who has a disability present. They want to be told in a private place with no disturbances, and to have adequate time for information to be given, questions asked, and further interviews scheduled.

When communication is handled in this way family

members tend to adapt more quickly and establish more positive relationships with each other, the person with the disability and professionals. However, many consultations with families are not conducted in this way, particularly initial diagnoses (Hornby, 1987). Many parents are angry and resentful about the way they were first told of the disability. This first, negative contact with a professional concerned with their family member who has a disability can sour their attitudes to future relationships with professionals. It therefore behoves all professionals to follow the above guidelines when communicating such information to parents or other family members.

Obtaining Information

One of the very first requests of family members, after receiving the diagnosis, is for comprehensive, accurate and up-to-date information about the person's handicapping condition (Philip and Duckworth, 1982). Most parents also want suggestions as to how they can facilitate the person's development. Families should also be told, at this time, about all the services and benefits available to help them care for their member with special needs. This information is widely available in the form of both written materials and professional expertise. It is therefore quite alarming to discover how often it does not get to the people who need it.

Receiving Support

Soon after the diagnosis family members need to have supportive counselling available to them. They need someone to help them express and clarify their feelings and to help in understanding their reactions and those of others around them (Furneaux, 1988). In this way families can be assisted to make a speedy and successful adaptation to the situation. If they do not receive such counselling, they may experience considerable anguish and take much longer to move through the adaptation process. However, people will seldom ask directly for counselling, whereas they will ask for information about the family member who has a disability. Therefore, it is important for the person who supplies family members with this information to also have the skills necessary to carry out supportive counselling (Gargiulo, 1985; Seligman, 1979).

Meeting Members of Other Exceptional Families

Surveys have shown that most parents want to meet others with children who have similar disabilities (Furneaux, 1988; Hornby, 1987). Whereas many parents wish to do this shortly after the diagnosis, some do not want such meetings for several months or even years. When parents do meet, they typically report great benefits both in terms of obtaining information and in receiving emotional support (Featherstone, 1981). Other family members, such as siblings and grandparents, also gain benefit from meeting with their peers from other exceptional families (Seligman and Darling, 1989). Professionals can help to facilitate these contacts by making families aware of the various support groups and other organizations operating in their area.

INDIVIDUAL, GROUP AND FAMILY INTERVENTIONS

Various interventions have emerged during recent years all with the aim of facilitating the development and functioning of families with members who have disabilities. Although each tends to focus on different members of the family, it is considered that all interventions can be conceived and carried out in a way that takes the entire family into account.

Counselling

As noted above, family members, including parents, siblings and grandparents, need to have counselling available to them from the time of diagnosis onwards. Therefore, in addition to having basic counselling skills sufficient to deal with everyday concerns, professionals must be able to refer family members on to qualified counsellors when the concerns raised would take them beyond their level of competence (Webster, 1977). With regard to parents, some feel more at ease in individual counselling

(Luterman, 1979), while others gain more from participation in group counselling sessions (Hornby and Singh, 1982). It is therefore important that professionals be aware of the various individuals and organizations in their community which can provide such counselling.

Training

Many parents of children with disabilities want to receive guidance from professionals in order to help them cope with their children's behaviour problems and facilitate their development (Harris, 1983; Topping, 1986). Such guidance, or parent training, can be organized individually, as in the Portage programme (White and Cameron, 1988) or in groups as with behavioural group training (Hornby and Singh, 1983). Group parent programmes can be designed to combine training with group counselling in order to provide a supportive environment in which parents can learn new skills and gain confidence through talking with other parents (Hornby and Murray, 1983). Likewise, it has been acknowledged that professionals involved in individual parent training should also combine it with the availability of counselling (Kaiser and Fox, 1986; Kroth, 1985; White and Cameron, 1988).

Two additional types of training programmes for parents have emerged recently. These are programmes to train parents in advocacy skills, and in coping skills (Schilling, 1988). In advocacy training parents are taught assertiveness skills in order to access services for people with disabilities, while in coping skills training parents are taught to develop their own personal coping strategies, social support networks, and community supports.

Workshops

The organization of workshops for parents of children with disabilities, in order to meet some of their counselling and training needs, was developed in the 1970s and is now well established (McConkey, 1985). More recently workshops have been developed in order to address the needs of other family members. The initial work was carried out as part of the Supporting Extended Family Members (SEFAM) project in Seattle in order to meet the needs of siblings, fathers, and grandparents.

'Sibshops' are workshops aimed at providing siblings of children with disabilities an opportunity to meet others in the same situation, to gain specific information on disabilities, and to learn how to handle common incidents which occur in exceptional families (Meyer, Vadasy and Fewell, 1985). The Fathers Programme also uses a workshop format so that fathers can discuss the emotional impact of the child's handicap on the family and learn activities and skills in order to be better able to facilitate their children's development (Meyer, Vadasy, Fewell and Schell, 1985). Grandparent Workshops offer opportunities for grandparents to meet each other as well as to obtain guidance from professionals on how best to provide support for the family (Vadasy, Fewell and Meyer, 1986).

Self-Help Groups

A major growth area in mental health services in recent years has been the proliferation of self-help groups (Gitterman and Shulman, 1986). Groups for families of people with disabilities have been no exception. In addition to the many groups for parents there are now organizations specifically for fathers, siblings and grandparents of people with disabilities. Each of these publishes a regular newsletter (see Fewell and Vadasy, 1986). One type of self-help group, which has shown quite rapid growth in numbers in recent years is the Parent to Parent Scheme. Parent to Parent services were first established in the U.S.A. and have subsequently spread to Canada, Australia, New Zealand and the U.K. (Hornby, 1988; McConkey, 1985). They are support services for parents of children with special needs in which support is provided by a team of volunteer parents who themselves have children with similar needs. Typically, Parent to Parent services operate as a telephone contact helpline. The Parent to Parent schemes in which the writer, and his colleagues, have been involved, have emphasized training parents in basic counselling skills (Hornby, Murray and Jones, 1987). Another feature of these schemes is that they include parents of children with a wide range of disabilities. This leads to links being established between parents of children who have different disabilities, and helps to break down the barriers which often exist between services for the groups with different disabilities.

Family Therapy

The application of family therapy principles and techniques (Fisch, Weakland and Segal, 1982; Minuchin and Fishman, 1981) to interventions with families of persons with disabilities is a most promising recent development. The family therapy literature provides the most comprehensive insight into how families are affected by interventions and how they change (Berger and Foster, 1986). By focusing on problems in the family structure or communication patterns, the dynamics of exceptional families can be better understood and therefore interventions designed in order to bring about constructive change in the functioning of the family as a whole. Apart from some notable exceptions (Berger, 1984; Coopersmith, 1984) little has been published to date on the use of family therapy with families of people with disabilities, but this type of intervention holds much promise for the future.

PROFESSIONAL ATTITUDES, KNOWLEDGE AND SKILLS

Clearly there is certain knowledge, attitudes and skills, over and above the expertise associated with each profession, which is needed in order to work effectively with people who have disabilities and their families.

Knowledge

Professionals should have a good understanding of the adaptation process and of the needs of parents and other family members. When parents react to events with anger, denial or sadness, professionals should be able to be non-defensive and to help them work through their feelings, and thereby progress to a mature emotional acceptance of the child and his or her disability. Professionals should also have a thorough knowledge of the dynamics of families of people with disabilities. This will enable interventions to be planned so that the functioning of such families is enhanced along with progress in the development of the person with the handicap.

Attitudes

The attitudes which professionals require in order to work effectively with families are ones which are consistent with the development of a productive partnership. To bring this about, professionals must possess the basic underlying attitudes of genuineness, respect and empathy (Rogers, 1980). They must be genuine in their relationships with members of the family. That is, they must come across as real people with strengths and weaknesses. For example, they should always be prepared to say that they 'don't know' when this is the case. In other words, they should relate to family members as people first and professionals second. Hiding behind a professional facade of competence is not in anyone's interest. Professionals should also show respect for family members of the person with a disability. Parents' opinions and requests should always be given the utmost consideration. In the final analysis parents' wishes must be respected even if they run counter to the views of professionals since it is they who have the long-term responsibility for the person who has a disability. Most importantly, professionals should try to develop empathy with family members. They should be able to see the situation from the point of view of the parents, siblings or grandparents. If professionals can develop an empathic understanding of the position of family members, then it is likely that a productive partnership will evolve.

Skills

In order to work effectively with families, professionals need good interpersonal communication skills. The most important part of this is the possession of basic counselling skills. Several authors have elaborated on the use of such skills with parents of children with special needs (Gargiulo, 1985; Seligman, 1979; Turnbull and Turnbull, 1986). Briefly, what is required is the ability to listen, understand, and help decide what action to take. Professionals must first of all listen to what family members have to say, in order to help them clarify their thoughts and feelings. They should then be helped to gain a clear understanding of the problem or concern which they have. Finally, professionals should help family members decide what, if anything, they want to do about their problem or concern – that is, what action they wish to take. Possessing the skills required to implement this simple three-step problem solving model of counselling will contribute enormously to the ability of professionals in establishing a productive working relationship with families.

CONCLUSION AND RECOMMENDATIONS

The most important variable in working with families of people with disabilities is the relationship which professionals establish. A positive, facilitative relationship is needed to promote a constructive working partnership. It is therefore important for professionals to develop a thorough understanding of the adaptation process and of the needs of family members for support and guidance. Professionals should also be familiar with various models of family functioning as applied to families of people with disabilities. They should also be aware of the range of interventions which can be used to meet the needs of such families. Most importantly, professionals should develop a high level of interpersonal communication skills including sound basic counselling skills. These skills will promote the establishment of productive working relationships with families, which will in turn facilitate the effectiveness of their intervention programmes with their clients who have disabilities.

Professionals need to:

1. Consider the families of people with disabilities when planning a treatment programme;

2. Develop a good understanding of the dynamics of such families, and of the process of adaptation likely to be experienced by their members;
3. Communicate the results of assessments and diagnostic tests in a sensitive and constructive manner;
4. Be able to give family members up-to-date information about the disability, and to help them express their concerns and feelings about its effects;
5. Ensure that families who care for members with disabilities receive all the benefits and services to which they are entitled;
6. Be aware of the potential stress on family members and be prepared to offer supportive counselling, or practical assistance, when necessary;
7. Recognize that the needs of individual family members may be different. For example, mothers may need more breaks from the constant care of the child who has a disability, fathers may need more help in coming to terms with the situation, and siblings may need to learn more about the disability;
8. Know of potential sources of help for such families such as: individual and group counselling; self-help groups; parent training; family therapy; and, workshops for parents, siblings or grandparents;
9. Be continually developing the specific knowledge, attitudes and skills necessary for achieving effective working relationships with people with disabilities and their families.

REFERENCES

Berger, M. (1984) 'Social Network Interventions for Families that have a Handicapped Child', in J.C. Hansen (ed), *Families with Handicapped Members*, Aspen, Rockville, MD.
Berger, M. and Foster, M. (1986) 'Applications of Family Therapy Theory to Research and Interventions with Families with Mentally Retarded Children', in J.J. Gallagher and P.M. Vietze (eds), *Families of Handicapped Persons: Research, Programs and Policy Issues*, Paul H.Brookes, Baltimore.
Blacher, J. (1984) 'Sequential Stages of Parental Adjustment to the

Birth of a Child with Handicaps: Fact or Artifact?', *Mental Retardation*, 22, 2, 55–68.

Bristol, M.M. and Gallagher, J.J. (1986) 'Research on Fathers of Young Handicapped Children', in J.J. Gallagher and P.M. Vietze (eds), *Families of Handicapped Persons*, Paul H. Brookes, Baltimore.

Brotherson, M.J., Turnbull, A.P., Summers, J.A. and Turnbull, H.R. (1986) 'Fathers of Disabled Children', in B.E. Robinson and R.L. Barret (eds), *The Developing Father*, Guilford, New York.

Bronfenbrenner, U. (1979) *The Ecology of Human Development* Harvard University Press, Cambridge, Mass.

Byrne, E.A., Cunningham, C.C. and Sloper, P. (1988) *Families and their Children with Down's Syndrome*, Routledge, London.

Chilman, C.S., Nunnally, E.W. and Cox, F.M. (eds) (1988) *Chronic Illness and Disability*, Sage, Newbury Park, CA.

Coopersmith, E.I. (ed) (1984) *Family Therapy with Families with Handicapped Children*, Aspen, Rockville, MD.

Crnic, K.A. and Leconte, J.M. (1986) 'Understanding Sibling Needs and Influences', in R.R. Fewell and P.F. Vadasy (eds), *Families of Handicapped Children*, Pro-Ed, Austin, Texas.

Featherstone, H. (1981) *A Difference in the Family*, Penguin, Harmondsworth.

Fewell, R.R. and Vadasy P.F. (eds) (1986) *Families of Handicapped Children*, Pro-Ed, Austin.

Fisch, R., Weakland, J. and Segal, L. (1982) *The Tactics of Change,* Jossey-Bass, San Francisco.

Furneaux, B. (1988) *Special Parents*, Open University Press, Milton Keynes.

Gargiulo, R.M. (1985) *Working with Parents of Exceptional Children,* Houghton Mifflin, Boston.

Gitterman, A. and Shulman, L. (eds) (1986) *Mutual Aid Groups and the Life Cycle* Peacock, Itasca, Il.

Harris, S.L. (1983) *Families of the Developmentally Disabled,* Pergamon, New York.

Hornby, G. (1987) 'Families with Exceptional Children', in D.R. Mitchell and N.N. Singh (eds), *Exceptional Children in New Zealand*, Dunmore Press, Palmerston North.

Hornby, G. (1988) 'Launching Parent to Parent Schemes', *British Journal of Special Education*, 15, 2, 77–78.

Hornby, G. and Murray, R. (1983) 'Group Programmes for Parents of Children with Various Handicaps', *Child: Care, Health and Development*, 9, 185–198.

Hornby, G., Murray, R. and Jones, R. (1987) 'Establishing a Parent to Parent Service', *Child: Care, Health and Development*, 13, 277–288.

Hornby, G. and Singh, N.N. (1982) 'Reflective Group Counselling for Parents of Mentally Retarded Children', *British Journal of Mental Subnormality, 28*, 71–76.

Hornby, G. and Singh, N.N. (1983) 'Group Training for Parents of Mentally Retarded Children', *Child: Care, Health and Development, 9*, 199–213.

Kaiser, A.P. and Fox, J.J. (1986) 'Behavioural Parent Training Research', in J.J. Gallagher and P.M. Vietze (eds) *Families of. Handicapped Persons*, Paul H. Brookes, Baltimore.

Kew, S. (1975) *Handicap and Family Crisis*, Pitman, London.

Kroth, R.L. (1985) *Communicating with Parents of Exceptional Children* (2nd ed), Love, Denver.

Lamb, M.E. (1983) 'Fathers of Exceptional Children', in M. Seligman (ed) *The Family with a Handicapped Child*, Grune and Stratton, New York.

Lonsdale, G. (1978) 'Family Life with a Handicapped Child: The Parents Speak', *Child: Care, Health and Development, 4*, 99–120.

Luterman, D. (1979) *Counselling Parents of Hearing Impaired Children*, Little Brown, New York.

Max, L. (1985) 'Parents' Views of Provisions, Services and Research', in N.N. Singh and K.N. Wilton (eds), *Mental Retardation in New Zealand*, Whitcoulls, Christchurch.

McConachie, H. (1986) *Parents and Young Mentally Handicapped Children: A Review of Research Issues*, Croom Helm, London.

McConkey, R. (1985) *Working with Parents*, Croom Helm, London.

Meyer, D.J. (1986) 'Fathers of Handicapped Children', in R.R. Fewell & P.F. Vadasy (eds), *Families of Handicapped Children*, Pro-Ed, Austin, TX.

Meyer, D.J., Vadasy, P.F. and Fewell, R.R. (1985) *Sibshops: A Handbook for Implementing Workshops for Siblings of Children with Special Needs*, University of Washington Press, Seattle.

Meyer, D.J., Vadasy, P.F., Fewell, R.R. and Schell, G.C. (1985) *A Handbook for the Fathers Program*, University of Washington Press, Seattle.

Minnes, P.M. (1988) 'Family Stress Associated with a Developmentally Handicapped Child', in N.W. Bray (ed) *International Review of Research in Mental Retardation* (vol. 15), Academic Press, London.

Minuchin, S. and Fishman, C. (1981) *Techniques of Family Therapy*, Harvard University Press, Cambridge.

Mitchell, D.R. (1985) 'Guidance Needs and Counselling of Parents of Persons with Intellectual Handicaps', in N.N. Singh and K.M.

Wilton (eds), *Mental Retardation in New Zealand*, Whitcoulls, Christchurch.

Murphy, M.A. (1982) 'The Family with a Handicapped Child: A Review of the Literature', *Developmental and Behavioural Pediatrics*, *3*, 73–82.

Olshansky, S. (1962) 'Chronic Sorrow: A Response to Having a Mentally Defective Child', *Social Casework*, 43, 190–193.

Philip, M. and Duckworth, D. (1982) *Children with Disabilities and Their Families: A Review of Research.* NFER-Nelson, Windsor.

Powell, T.H. and Ogle, P.A. (1985) *Brothers and Sisters: A Special Part of Exceptional Families*, Paul H. Brookes, Baltimore.

Rogers, C.R. (1980) *A Way of Being*, Houghton Mifflin, Boston.

Sameroff, A.J. and Chandler, M.J. (1975) 'Reproductive Risk and the Continuum of Caretaking Casualty', in F.D. Horowitz (ed), *Review of Child Development Research* (vol. 4), University of Chicago Press, Chicago.

Seligman, M. (1979) *Strategies for Helping Parents of Exceptional Children*, Free Press, New York.

Seligman, M. and Darling, R.B. (1989) *Ordinary Families, Special Children: A Systems Approach to Childhood Disability*, Guilford, New York.

Schilling, R. F. (1988) 'Helping Families with Developmentally Delayed Members', in C.S. Chilman, E.W. Nunnally and F.M. Cox (eds), *Chronic Ilness and Disability*, Sage, Newbury Park.

Simeonsson, R. J. and McHale, S. (1981) 'Review: Research on Handicapped Children: Sibling Relationships', *Child: Care, Health and Development*, 7, 153 - 171

Sonnek, I.M. (1986) 'Grandparents and the Extended Family of Handicapped Children', in R.R. Fewell and P.V. Vadasy (eds), *Families of Handicapped Children*, Pro-Ed, Austin, TX.

Topping, K.J. (1986) *Parents as Educators*, Croom Helm, London.

Turnbull, A.P., Summers, J.A. and Brotherson, M.J. (1984) *Working with Families with Disabled Members*, University of Kansas, Kansas.

Turnbull, A.P. and Turnbull, H.R. (1986) *Families, Professionals and Exceptionality*, Merrill, Columbus.

Vadasy, P.F., Fewell, R.R. and Meyer, D.J. (1986) 'Grandparents of Children with Special Needs: Insights into their Experiences and Concerns', *Journal of the Division for Early Childhood*, *10*,1, 36 - 44.

Webster, E.J. (1977) *Counselling with Parents of Handicapped Children*, Grune and Stratton, New York.

White, M. and Cameron, R.J. (eds) (1988) *Portage: Progress, Problems and Possibilities*, NFER-Nelson, Windsor.

Wikler, L. (1981) 'Chronic Stresses in Families of Mentally Retarded Children', *Family Relations*, 30, 281–288.

Wikler, L. (1986) 'Periodic Stresses of Families of Older Mentally
    Retarded Children: An Exploratory Study', *American Journal
    of Mental Deficiency, 90*, 703–706.
Wikler, L., Wasow, M. and Hatfield, E. (1981) 'Chronic Sorrow
    Revisited', *American Journal of Orthopsychiatry, 51*, 63–70.
Wright, J.S., Granger, R.D. and Sameroff, A.J. (1984) 'Parental
    Acceptance and Developmental Handicap', in J. Blacher (ed),
    Severely Handicapped Young Children and Their Families,
    Academic Press, Orlando.

Chapter Eight

DISABILITY COUNSELLING: GRIEVING THE LOSS

Susan B. Webb

INTRODUCTION

In this chapter the importance of addressing grieving processes is considered particularly as it concerns the counsellor working with people who have disabilities. We all recognize the role of grief in coming to terms with losses, in fact it has been the subject of extensive academic and popular self-help literature. However, little writing on grieving deals in any detail with losses resulting from disabilities, and conversely literature on disability largely ignores the importance of grieving for and by people with disabilities.

The idea developed here is that grief follows *inevitably* from disability. Atkins, Lynch and Pullo (1982) describe 'disability' as a condition of impairment, physical or mental, having an objective aspect that can usually be medically described. Bowlby (1969, 1973) sees grief as the sequence of subjective experiences that result from mourning, and mourning to mean the range of behavioural and psychological consequences resulting from loss. All disability involves loss and if grieving is not experienced, then it will be hard for other, more obvious, gains to be made. There is the real danger that potential abilities will not be developed fully, if at all.

Losses may be multi-faceted, some visible, some invisible, some apparent, some symbolic. Some will only arise at a time long after the person acquires a disability, while others will be immediately obvious.

The moment of loss itself does not have to have been experienced directly by the client, as for instance when problems develop before or at birth. Even though people have not experienced possessing what is lost, it is still felt as a loss, because they recognize that they differ from what might be commonly regarded as 'normal'.

Grieving for all persons, including those with disabilities, is thus a complex process which may return at various lifestages as the different aspects of a loss become important. Grief may need to be experienced many times, not in order to repeat past feelings but to rework them in a new context or deal with the loss from a new angle. The counsellor, therefore, needs to be aware of not only the commonly accepted developmental stages of the grieving process, but also the way in which different aspects of the loss may be experienced at various stages. Furthermore, the counsellor needs to be aware that losses may have different meanings, each of which may need addressing at different times over a person's life-span.

The task for counsellors is to provide the right climate for grieving. They need to bear in mind that much of this process is experienced quite naturally by people with disabilities, both within themselves and in the contexts in which they live, such as their families. The counsellor's task is only to facilitate a normal process, if that is necessary, and to help clients with disabilities address the relevant issues if they have difficulty moving on from a particular point. Once appropriate grieving strategies are developed, people find it much easier to work through further grief without extra assistance.

In this chapter the relationship of grief to disability, grief and the individual with a disability, and the family and their grief are considered. The counsellor's response to grief and strategies for counselling are then outlined.

GRIEF AND DISABILITY

Bowlby's definition, cited earlier, relates grief and mourning to loss of an attachment object, either a person or an actual object. Werner-Beland (1980) postulates that, in adult life, an important attachment object is the self. Thus damage or loss in relation to the self may be taken to mean the loss of part of an attachment object. Bailey and Gregg (1986) see loss through bodily injury as comparable to the loss of a loved one through death, but it must be remembered that where death is final, the nature of a person's disability may change over time. Grieving is regarded as a normal developmental process, involving stages (Kubler-Ross, 1969, 1974) through which a person works. At times, however, a person becomes overwhelmed, or arrested at a particular point in the process, or maladaptive behaviour emerges. These are often regarded as forms of pathological grief (Bailey and Gregg, 1986). Counsellors should be cautious about identifying grief as pathological, thus giving it a negative and illness-oriented label. Normal grieving also includes times when the grieving process does not progress. Behaviours and attitudes that might be defined as pathological may just be indicative of an unexplored aspect of the loss, not yet integrated into feeling and thinking.

Just as western societies have become increasingly inept at handling death and dying, so has their addressing of grief in other situations. Bailey and Gregg (1986) point out that we have no ritualized process for dealing with losses associated with a disability, increasing the risk of pathological grieving. Invisible losses, such as infertility, are especially difficult in this respect. Counsellors need to remember, however, that cultures may interpret losses differently and have their own ways of grieving for them, just as they may view the disability itself differently (Percic, 1986).

It is also important to recognize that a sense of loss may be felt, and therefore grieved, even if the moment of loss has never been experienced, or the lost function used. Although Simos (1979) argues that loss (having had and then not having) differs from deprivation (having never had), it remains true that people live in a social context and are aware of how they might have expected to be. This loss of potential is as much to be struggled with and mourned as any experienced loss.

Losses through disablement involve complex grief. Whereas the major experience of loss through death occurs at the time of loss, and further grieving is mainly experienced as an echo of the first grief, the impact of loss may be considerably delayed in disability and, as Werner-Beland (1980) states, there is no foreseeable end to grief or its closure. In bereavement the process of grieving can be largely completed, but in disability the losses remain an integral part of daily life. While the bereaved person must learn to close the gap left by the dead, the person with a disability must learn to live with the gap left by the disability.

It is helpful to interpret the various suggested stages of grieving in a broad sense. Just as dying patients and their families do not progress in an orderly manner from stage to stage, but return from time to time to other stages, so in disability counselling progress will also not be straightforward. The actual stages of grieving will be considered in more detail later in this chapter.

A developmental perspective on the grief of a person with a disability posits that at different times the gap left by the loss will have different meanings, according to age and life stage. Aspects of the loss which have been known and perhaps apparently accepted because at the time they were not important, re-emerge as unresolved grief when they become significant. Disabling conditions may also be progressive and each new development brings with it not only the need to resolve the new loss but also a reactivation of previous unresolved feelings (Bailey and Gregg, 1986).

Losses are also symbolic. Physical loss may be experienced as a step towards one's own death (Werner-Beland, 1980; Bailey and Gregg, 1986). The person has lost his or her prior concept of self (Bailey and Gregg, 1986) and sense of continuity with that self. At the same time he or she is struggling with the social impact of what the condition may symbolize to others.

Thus grieving the loss may be a complex and recurring process in disability, which requires particular patience and sensitivity on the part of a counsellor. Different aspects of the loss may surface at various stages of the person's life. Also several stages in the grieving process may be evident at the same time as different aspects of the loss are worked through separately. We will now look at what this may mean for the person who has a disability.

GRIEF AND THE INDIVIDUAL WITH A DISABILITY

As has been discussed already, grieving the loss is an important part of coming to terms with disability. Each loss will have many facets, concrete and symbolic, visible and invisible, and recognizing each of these and coming to terms with them is likely to be gradual. Grieving is a natural process through which individuals work and, for the most part, the tasks will be achieved without outside help. At times, however, a little assistance is useful in quickening the process or in assisting the person who has become blocked or overwhelmed.

To begin with, it can be difficult for the person with a disability to feel he or she has the right to grieve. Grief responses are often ignored by health professionals (Werner-Beland, 1980) as they focus on the physical care and repair of the person. What is more, the exact extent of the loss may not be clear at the time of the initial crisis. The person who has recently incurred a disability may be unsure, for some considerable time, as to how much he or she needs to grieve. Possible advances in medical technology can make it unclear whether present loss of functions should be grieved or not.

In cases where the client is hospitalized as an immediate result of acquiring a disability, particular care needs to be taken, since the focus of hospital staff is frequently on getting the patient well enough to leave and not on addressing the changed quality of life of the person. However, the emotional component of the problem may be sufficient to prevent the patient from becoming independent and resuming previous social roles (Watson, 1985). Viney and Benjamin (1983) suggest that interaction in hospital can actually foster helplessness in response to crisis. Bailey and Gregg (1986) discuss the use of a linking object by a bereaved person to represent the deceased and state that this is a symptom of pathological grief. Reluctance by a person who has a disability to move on from a particular hospital context, stage of recovery or piece of equipment may also result from a desire to maintain contact with the lost function.

The need to grieve may be masked behind a determination to improve. There is a popularly held belief that positive thinking is an important tool for healing and recovery. It therefore becomes very easy to think that feelings of sadness, depression, anger and helplessness are unhelpful. However, unresolved grief is a form of stress, and as such, without being resolved, will undermine the value of positive thinking. Stress has been noted as depleting a person of physical energy and can also precipitate physical disorders, increase pain and aggravate existing difficulties (Goodwin and Holmes, 1988).

Kubler-Ross' (1969) description of the stages of grieving: shock and denial, anger, bargaining, depression and acceptance, have been much discussed and various writers have provided alternative structures (Davenport, 1981; Seguine, 1985; Simos, 1979; Worden, 1982). These mainly seem to break down Kubler-Ross' stages into a larger number of sub-sets, or to reorganize the order of stages. Hers remain a simpler and, therefore, probably more useful tool for the practitioner to track the progress of grief-work. We need to bear in mind, however, that people will not move neatly from stage to stage and that, because grieving is a complex process, they may approach stages in a different order and may appear to move backwards and forwards between some stages.

There is a parallel description of stages in literature on adjustment to disability (cf. Livneh and Evans, 1984). Reichart and MacGuffie (1988) describe adjusting to AIDS as involving an initial crisis which includes denial and overwhelming anxiety, early adjustment, acceptance and preparation for death. These link with some of Kubler-Ross' stages. Viney and Benjamin (1983) see anxiety, depression, helplessness and social isolation as responses to a crisis period in hospital. These symptoms seem to relate more to the depression phase. Werner-Beland (1980) suggests that phases of grief evolve in correspondence to stages of physical recovery and rehabilitation and this notion fits with a developmental approach to grieving. While Reichart and MacGuffie (1988) claim that emotional regression occurs sometimes in the acceptance phase, this may be perceived as experiencing the loss from a new perspective and Werner-Beland (1980) suggests that grief reappears when illness or disability become conspicuous once more, or interfere with a new goal achievement. Goodwin and Holmes (1988) also point out that grief may appear as a result of new losses which would not have occurred without the prior existence of the disability, for instance when people with disabilities are the victims of violent crime and experience their vulnerability to unwarranted attack. It is worth examining how the stages may be exhibited.

> An adolescent girl whose mother was infected by rubella during early pregnancy was confronted with the fact that both her limited sight and hearing were deteriorating further. Her initial reaction was to ignore the problem, refusing to visit the appropriate specialists, despite encouragement from

her teachers. When the situation could be avoided no longer, she moved into very angry functioning with her family, peers and teachers; the 'why me' stage. She was particularly angry with her younger sister who was at the same grade level as her. This stage was very difficult as her anger was quite violent, probably as a result of her parents' difficulties in listening to her anger in the past. Bargaining consisted of a series of unrealistic views on how to remedy the situation; if her class mates could only be quieter, if she could rest her eyes more, if only she didn't need to study at night. Depression followed. It seemed pointless to continue with her schooling, she was already considerably older than her classmates, her parents did not understand and the necessary new equipment was impossible to use. Finally, acceptance was reached and she realized that there need be no shame attached to her slowed academic career, that her career goals were still achievable, and that parents and other adults were sympathetic to her problems.

Loss may involve different meanings at different life stages. A man, as a young boy, became confined to a wheelchair as a result of spinal cord injury in a motor accident. Initial losses included the ability to participate in his peer group's activities, some independence and bodily control, and previously enjoyed sporting activities. During adolescence he had to face his loss of 'normal' attractiveness to girls, worries about his sexuality, his inability to be indistinguishable in a group, and difficulties to do with learning to drive a motor vehicle and all that that symbolized. As a young adult, career options were reduced and travel more difficult to manage. As the parent of young children he grieved his inability to play with his children as other fathers could. Later in life he may suffer reduced mobility and may develop physical problems resulting from additional stresses placed on certain parts of his body.

People with disabilities need to be allowed to grieve their

losses. This is not always easy given the major focus on rehabilitation in treatment settings. Sound rehabilitation is unlikely, however, without this process. Shock and denial, anger, bargaining and depression are likely to be experienced before acceptance is reached. Grieving is complicated by the many facets of the losses and by progression through developmental stages in the lifespan.

GRIEF AND THE FAMILY

As can be seen from the examples above, people with a disability do not exist in a vacuum, but must live out their difficulties in relation to others, particularly those who are emotionally significant to them. Family members are not only important to the individual's resolution of grief but must also struggle with their own grief reactions to the loved-one's loss.

Families as units appear to work through the same stages of grieving as individuals (Hendrich, 1981). Bray (1977) describes adjustment stages of fear, denial, anger, depression and acceptance and Sutton (1985) suggests that family adjustment may be difficult because it is similar and parallel to that of the person with the disability. Moreover, children, in particular, may feel inappropriately responsible for a parent's accident. Goodwin and Holmes (1988) point out that when a person who has a disability is later the victim of crime and suffers additional loss, the family may also be grieving and unable to provide help and support.

Conversely, some family experience will be different; the losses, although based on the same set of events, are not the same. For instance, the parents of a young adult, injured in a swimming accident mourned the loss of their newly acquired freedom from a full-time parenting role. A man who had been responsible through negligence for his accident at work felt guilty, while his wife was angry with him and felt reluctant to care for him. Family members may feel they have no right to grieve for themselves, when the losses of a person with a disability are so much greater than their own.

If family members and the individual are in different stages of grieving, they can be of little assistance to each other. If the individual is struggling with anger about the loss and the family are still denying that it will have a significant impact on family life, there is little room for open and constructive communication.

Families may also grieve in anticipation of certain events, in order to protect themselves and the person who has a disability from later sadness. This may not be appropriate for the individual. A young woman who had been a polio victim as a baby had been brought up to believe that she stood little chance of ever marrying, that it would probably be impossible for her to bear children, although there was no medical evidence to support this, and that her career options were seriously limited. During adolescence she was confused as to whether these aspects were to be mourned or not. By her late twenties, however, she had studied overseas, trained and taught as a teacher of maladjusted children, married and had two small children of her own.

There is, however, a recognized role for the family in achieving adjustment for the person with a disability (Buscaglia, 1975), but this can only be of use if the family members themselves are able to adjust. Evans, Halar and Bishop (1986) found that family involvement was helpful in achieving treatment compliance from stroke victims. The cultural mores of a family will be important in mobilizing help. For instance in cultures based on multi-generational extended families, it is common for older family members to provide advice and solve problems (Percic, 1986).

Counsellors need to be aware of the likely impact of disabilities on family dynamics. From systems theory (cf. Barker, 1986) we know that factors, which may have been produced by events external to the family, become incorporated in family emotional life, and both cause and react to other issues in the family. Therefore even if a person who has a disability works at coming to terms with losses, this may not be sufficient if the family too have not resolved their grief. The family may insist that the problem does not exist, or may express inappropriate anger towards helping professionals, which interferes with the progress of treatment. Parents may expend energy on unrealistic campaigns to improve provisions for their child, which deprive the child of valuable ordinary parenting time.

If there are pre-existing difficulties within the family, then the disability may be incorporated inappropriately into family functioning as a way of maintaining 'homeostasis', the existing state of balance between parts of the family system. For instance, the parents of a child with a disability promoted an unhelpful level of dependence in the child because it enabled them to ignore marital difficulties unconnected with the loss.

Just as the loss for the individual who has a disability will have different meanings at different life stages, so will the loss have different meanings for family members according to the stage of their own development. As stages change, family members too must adapt to new aspects of the loss. Children of an adult who has a disability may mourn, in childhood, the loss of a physically active parent. In middle age they may mourn the loss of separateness for their own nuclear family resulting from care for the parent.

To summarize, family grief is therefore as much to be expected as individual grief. Grief will progress through stages, and aspects of the loss will be grieved at different times according to life-stages. Just as individuals work naturally through the grief process, so do families. They may, however, need the counsellor to facilitate this process at times and to encourage communication of the grief to other family members, including the person who has a disability. Where a family finds it difficult to move beyond a particular stage, or where the disability is being used to avoid confronting other family problems, then it would be wise for family therapy to be undertaken.

GRIEF, DISABILITY AND THE COUNSELLOR

Counsellors need to deal with their reactions both to grief and to disability. Reichart and MacGuffie (1988), discussing the role of the AIDS counsellor, suggest that it is extremely important for counsellors to deal with their own feelings about the syndrome. They may, however, also be hampered by unresolved grief of their own that in no concrete manner relates to the grief of the person with the disability. In order for counsellors to feel at ease in the presence of those who are grieving they have to be comfortable with their own grief. Heikkenen (1981) contends that the failure of counsellors to work on their own loss may be the biggest block to client change.

Counsellors also may feel guilty for not having a disability themselves or for being 'luckier' than their clients. Since this is a feeling that will be shared by others in the context in which the person with a disability moves, it is extremely important for counsellors to be clear about this aspect of themselves and not allow it to intrude on their work.

Their own feelings of powerlessness and inadequacy in the face of the crisis confronting the person with a disability may also be an issue. These feelings are likely to reflect similar ones in the person who has a disability at the time. Such feelings in the counsellor often relate to a fear that there is nothing they can 'do' to help the person, when in fact what is required is simply being oneself. When we feel inadequate in relation to achieving any significant difference for our client, it is often difficult to recognize the much greater power of our being there and available to listen. While Stewart (1979) points out that counsellors need to be able to provide information, not just counselling, it is also important to differentiate between what is the client's need for information and the counsellor's need to feel useful. Focusing on what may be solved, rather than on the emotional pain, may well help the counsellor to feel less powerless, but in fact will do little to facilitate ultimate adjustment for the client.

Counsellors may experience particular difficulty with client's anger. They need to recognize this anger as an indication of the level of fear at having lost control of life. During angry stages clients may behave unpleasantly to nearly all those who come into contact with them. The resulting sense of isolation only worsens the anger. Counsellors need to be comfortable with encouraging the expression of anger towards themselves and with allowing anger towards others, however unreasonable it may seem, to be discussed. Not only the person with the disability but his or her family also may need to express anger. As a representative of the 'helping professions', counsellors may need to accept anger that belongs with other caregivers, who may be less able to handle it.

Counsellors also need to take particular care of themselves. Stav, Florian and Shuka (1986) state that those working with people with disabilities are under the same sort of pressure as those working with bereaved families and that this pressure can cause burnout. Personal involvement is inevitable and the risk of burnout is greater with 'chronic' clients who are involved with the counsellor over long periods, and who show no sign of improvement. They also state that the use of supervision is linked with lower rates of burnout. In supervision, counsellors can explore their own reactions to their clients' difficulties and address unresolved grief of their own, as well as looking in a more objective way at what is likely to be happening for their clients and their clients' families.

In summary, this section underlines the importance of counsellor self-awareness and ease with self. Counsellors need to be able to trust their 'being' as well as their 'doing' selves in relation to clients. While helping clients to solve problems is obviously an important part of their role, they must recognize that they may be able to listen to clients' distress in a way that others involved in helping them cannot.

COUNSELLING STRATEGIES

While it is the self that the counsellor brings to the counselling that matters most to the client, there are still useful strategies for the counsellor to be aware of when working with grieving clients. Underpinning these, however, is the need for a preparedness to address whatever the client raises and a recognition of the importance of being with the client while she or he expresses difficult feelings, rather than looking for ways to feel helpful. The counsellor also needs to be aware of the whole person, not just the presenting disability. Stewart (1979) reminds us that a person with a handicap is a person, not a handicap.

The setting for counselling is always important. While it may be difficult in some cases to obtain complete privacy, this is highly desirable, even in a hospital setting. Enough time needs to be allowed and a lack of interruptions arranged. The counsellor needs to remember that it may be more difficult for persons with disabilities to terminate the counselling session of their own accord and be sensitive to messages to do so.

Certain basic attending behaviours can enhance counsellor effectiveness (cf. Egan, 1986). Eye contact needs to be natural, and the counsellor should sit facing the client, if possible at the same height. These may not always be easy to achieve with clients who have disabilities, but as far as possible need to be incorporated. Where any particular behaviour is problematic, the counsellor may need to use others to compensate. For instance, when working with the sight-impaired, additional non-verbal encouragers and touch may need to be used to convey empathy, in order to compensate for the lack of eye-contact.

Non-verbal communication from client to counsellor may be restricted or altered and particularly when intense feelings, such as grief, are being expressed, nonverbal communication becomes critical. The counsellor needs to take into account the nature of the disability and be sensitive to the particular ways in which the individual is able to convey such information.

Clients need to be allowed to progress at their own pace through their grief. Trying to convince a client who is in the denial stage that it would be helpful to be angry, or an angry one that acceptance is the preferred goal, is not only a waste of the counsellor's time, but potentially a very destructive experience for the client, since it threatens what may be very fragile defenses. Counsellors should never collude with clients in ignoring the severity of the situation, but they should not force unwelcome information on them either.

While many different counselling approaches may be helpful and all counsellors operate with those with which they are most comfortable, some approaches offer particular strengths for grief counselling, especially where they focus on the exploration of feelings. Watson (1985) suggests that the counselling interventions used in her study of surgical patients were effective because exploration was what the clients required.

Thurer (1985) claims that psychodynamic theory offers a developmental perspective on reactions to disability and that psychodynamic therapists were the first to address issues of loss and grief. She sees this approach as particularly suited to dealing with losses in physical functioning and associated symbolic losses. Moreover, the counsellor may use understanding of the concept of transference to recognize parallels between the client's feelings towards the counsellor and significant others, and counter-transference to understand feelings that the client may be eliciting in others.

Gestalt therapy, with its emphasis on 'unfinished business', also offers a useful framework for working through grief (Allen, 1985). Gestalt dialogues may be used to explore the relationships between able and disabled parts of the client and gestalt fantasy may enable lost functions to be farewelled.

Werner-Beland (1980) recommends that intrapsychic, interpersonal and socio-economic losses should all be taken into account. This suggests the addition of a systems approach to what is described above. This would help the client to look at the impact of losses on close relationships and on the wider social context.

Counselling with the whole family (Hendrich, 1981) may also be appropriate in order to open up communication and express grief. Counsellors should take care not to become involved in discussing the feelings experienced by the person who has a disability with the family in her or his absence, and vice versa. Open communication needs to be fostered directly between family members. Families need to be able to function without the counsellor as an additional member of the family system and communication between two people about a third may create unhelpful triangles (Bowen, 1978). Systemic family therapy (cf. Selvini Palazzoli, Boscolo, Cecchin & Parata, 1978) advocates the setting of rituals; formalized shared tasks to recognize endings and herald beginnings. Given the invisibility of some losses and consequent difficulty in mourning them, this strategy may be of great value. It is also suggested that support groups for families (Sutton, 1985) and self-help groups (Reichart and MacGuffie, 1988) may be useful.

Counsellors need to be aware of cultural meanings and be sensitive to cultural differences. Aspects of loss may differ in their significance and grief may be expressed in unfamiliar ways. In addition, helping networks may function differently from culture to culture and family responses may not conform to those expected by the counsellor. Clients themselves are the best source of information for counsellors on these matters.

This section has looked briefly at a number of strategies that may be useful in disability counselling where grief is at issue. While all counsellors will operate within the frameworks dictated by their own inclinations and taught them in their training, certain approaches offer points of particular value in resolving the losses associated with disability.

CONCLUSION

This chapter has considered the role of the counsellor in resolving grief issues associated with loss in the context of disabilities. It is contended that grief is a developmental process which possesses stages and in that it is linked to development through the life-span. The resolution of grief is a complex process, with different stages of grieving being evident at any one time in relation to various aspects of the loss. Also, grief may reappear when a person moves into a new developmental stage and losses become significant in new ways.

Counsellors need to address grief issues for both individuals and families as they arise. Clients and their families should not be forced to function at stages which they have not reached and should be allowed to progress at their own pace, with the counsellor acting primarily as facilitator. In particular, open communication about grief between family members is important.

Counsellors should consider issues that concern their own functioning too. Self awareness and the ability to cope with both their own grief and that of others are important. Supervision is of great importance in achieving this.

All frameworks which enable the resolution of grief will be useful to the counsellor, but psychodynamic, gestalt and family therapy offer particular opportunities for the counsellor. Counsellors need to be aware that it is the extent to which they are able to be 'with' the client that is of the greatest significance.

For clients, the early acquisition of appropriate grieving skills will provide coping strategies which they will be able to use again, and which, in turn, will help them to assist others in the resolution of their grief. Conversely, without the strategies to resolve grief, other gains may simply never be achieved. Unlike the bereaved, clients with disabilities are obliged to live intimately with their losses for the rest of their lives. Such close contact demands the most constructive relationship possible.

RECOMMENDATIONS FOR COUNSELLING

This section lists the major points for counsellors discussed in the text of this chapter.

1. Grief is a natural, though complex, process and counsellors should follow their clients' pace through its stages.
2. The client needs the counsellor's 'being' rather than 'doing' self.

3. Counsellors should be alert to the possibility of grief being reactivated in response to different meanings to the loss over time.
4. It is appropriate for clients to grieve, even if the moment of loss has not been experienced (as with birth defects).
5. Grief may be masked by helplessness or, conversely, a determination to improve.
6. Counsellors should be sensitive to cultural difference in relation to grieving.
7. Counselllors should recognize their own feelings of guilt, grief, helplessness and inadequacy, and use their supervision to address these.
8. Counsellors need to be aware that non–verbal communication may be restricted or altered.
9. Psychodynamic, gestalt and systems frameworks are especially suited to grief work.
10. The grief of family members will differ from that of the client who has a disability, even though grieving the same event.
11. Open communication amongst family members about feelings associated with the disability is particularly valuable.
12. Counsellors should consider the impact of a disability on family dynamics, and realize that it may feed into existing inappropriate family functioning.
13. Family counselling may help reduce triangulation and facilitate family recognition of the loss.
14. Support groups may be of assistance to families.

REFERENCES

Allen, H.A. (1985) 'The Gestalt Perspective', *Journal of Applied Rehabilitation Counseling, 16*, 3, 21–25.
Atkins, B., Lynch, R. and Pullo, R. (1982) 'A Definition of Psychosocial Aspects of Disability: A Synthesis of the Literature', *Vocational Evaluation and Work Adjustment Bulletin, Summer,* 55–62.
Bailey, B. and Gregg, C. (1986) 'Grief, Pathological Grief and Rehabilitation Counseling', *Journal of Applied Rehabilitation Counseling, 17*, 4, 19–23.
Barker, P. (1986) *Basic Family Therapy*, (2nd ed,) Collins, London.
Bowen, M. (1978) *Family Therapy in Clinical Practice*, Jason Aronson New York.

Bowlby, J. (1969) *Attachment and Loss, Vol 1: Attachment.* Basic Books Inc., New York.

Bowlby, J. (1973) *Attachment and Loss, Vol. 2: Separation, Anxiety and Anger*, Basic Books Inc., New York.

Bray, G. (1977) 'Reactive Patterns in Families of the Severely Disabled', *Rehabilitation Counseling Bulletin*, 20, 236–239.

Buscaglia, L. (1975) *The Disabled and Their Parents: A Counseling Challenge*, Charles B. Slack Inc., New Jersey.

Davenport, D. (1981) 'A Closer Look at the "Healthy" Grieving Process', *Personnel and Guidance Journal*, 59, 6, 332–334.

Egan, G. (1986) *The Skilled Helper: A Systematic Approach to Effective Helping* (3rd ed), Brooks/Cole Publishing Co., Monterey.

Evans, R., Halar, E. and Bishop, D. (1986) 'Family Function and Treatment Compliance After Stroke', *International Journal of Rehabilitation Research*, 9, 1, 70–72.

Goodwin, L. and Holmes, G. (1988) 'Counseling the Crime Victim: A Guide for Rehabilitation Counselors', *International Journal of Rehabilitation Research*, 9, 1, 70–72.

Heikkenen, C. (1981) 'Loss Resolution and Growth', *Personnel and Guidance Journal*, 59, 6, 327–331.

Hendrich, S.S. (1981) 'Spinal Cord Injury: A Special Kind of Loss', *Personnel and Guidance Journal*, 59, 6, 355–359.

Kubler-Ross, E. (1969) *On Death and Dying.*, MacMillan, New York.

Livneh, H. and Evans, J. (1984) 'Adjusting to Disability: Behavioural Correlates and Intervention Strategies', *Personnel and Guidance Journal*, 62, 6, 363–365.

Percic, J.M. (1986) 'Cultural Factors and Rehabilitation Counseling;', *Journal of Applied Rehabilitation Counseling*, 17, 1, 52–53.

Reichart, D. & MacGuffie, R. (1988) 'A.I.D.S.: An Overview for Rehabilitation Counselors', *Journal of Applied Rehabilitation Counseling*, 19, 2, 34–37.

Seguine, A. (1985) 'The Psychology of Dying: A Redefinition of the Five Stages', in O. Margolis, H. Raether, A. Kutscher, A. Klagsbrun, E. Marcus, V. Pine and D. Cherico (eds), *Loss, Grief and Bereavement: A Guide for Counseling.* Praegar Publishers, New York.

Selvini Palazzoli, M., Boscolo, L., Cecchin, G. and Parata, G. (1978) *Paradox and Counterparadox*, Jason Aronson, New York.

Simos, B. (1979) *A Time to Grieve: Loss as a Universal Human Experience*, Family Service Association of America.

Stav A., Florian, V. and Shuka, E. (1986) 'Burnout Among Social Workers Working with Physically Disabled and Bereaved Families', *Journal of Social Science Research*, 10, 1, 81–94.

Stewart, W. (1979) *The Sexual Side of Handicap: A Guide for the Caring Professions*, Woodhead-Faulkner, Cambridge.

Sutton, J. (1985) 'The Need for Family Involvement in Client Rehabilitation', *Journal of Applied Rehabilitation Counseling*, 16, 1, 42–45.

Thurer, S. (1985) 'Rehabilitation Counseling: A Psychodynamic Perspective', *Journal of Applied Rehabilitation Counseling*, 16, 3, 4–8.

Viney, L. and Benjamin, Y. (1983) 'A Hospital-based Counseling Service for Medical and Surgical Patients', *Journal of Applied Rehabilitation Counseling*, 14, 2, 29–34.

Watson, P. (1985) 'Post-operative Counseling in Surgical Acute Care Settings: A Role for the Rehabilitation Counselor', *Journal of Applied Rehabilitation Counseling*, 16, 1, 36–38.

Werner-Beland, J. (1980) *Grief Responses to Long-Term Illness and Disability*, Reston Publishing Co. Inc., Virginia.

Worden, W. (1982) *Grief Counseling and Grief Therapy*. Springer Publishing Co., New York.

Chapter Nine

COUNSELLING PEOPLE WHO ARE UNEMPLOYED

Michael J. Holosko

INTRODUCTION

For the most part, the western industrialized world took the meaning of work for granted up until the post-Industrial Revolution and the Great Depression of 1929. After this time, the political-economic structures of industry, commerce, and government, as well as the academic world, including economists, sociologists, and psychologists, began to direct their attention toward the meaning of work and unemployment to society as a whole (Beales and Lambert, 1934; Beveridge, 1930; Krafchik, 1985), and the implications of work and unemployment for individuals (Bakke, 1934; Ginzburg, 1943; Liem and Rayman, 1982; O'Brien, 1985). There has been a plethora of empirical and theoretical research directed toward the former issue (i.e., the macro societal interpretations of work and unemployment), and a dearth of literature and information about the latter (i.e., how work and unemployment affects individuals).

It would not be a gross over-generalization to suggest that in most of Europe, Great Britain, the USA and Canada, unemployment is a profound reality which affects the lives of millions of persons. Indeed, whichever national data or statistical source one examines from the western world, the bottom line is that unemployment is ubiquitous and escalating in a steadily incremental pattern. This fact has some economists legitimately worried as they are unable to predict accurately the statistical estimates of these parameters (Haveman and Wolfe,

1984; Johnson, 1983; Perry, 1972). This has social and behavioural scientists concerned as it is a growing and prevalent societal problem which does not seem to be "curable" (Reigle, 1982). A review of the literature on unemployment clearly suggests that it seems to be running rampant with no end in sight, and there is not much we can do about it.

Despite this, it is important for those interested in rehabilitation counselling to understand issues related to helping this growing group of persons in society. This chapter provides an overview of various issues related to counselling those who are unemployed and considers the implications and commonalities with those who have disabilities. As the reader will note, however, the principles of counselling described herein are relevant to social workers, vocational counsellors and a variety of helping professionals (e.g., mental health counsellors, rehabilitation counsellors, and family service practitioners).

Two assumptions lay the foundation for this chapter. The first is that the information presented is directed towards micro counselling or direct practice with individuals, small groups, or families. The second is that although clients who come into counselling may be "something else" and unemployed (e.g., deaf and unemployed, mentally handicapped and unemployed, depressed and unemployed), the main presenting problem confronting the counsellor is that the client is unemployed. Thus, the primary role of the counsellor is directed towards the assessment and intervention of the unemployment problem. The chapter is organized according to:

1. The uniqueness of being unemployed;
2. The client-in-context;
3. Implications for practice.

THE UNIQUENESS OF BEING UNEMPLOYED

First off, let's not fool ourselves about trying to simplify an understanding of what it is truly like for a person to be unemployed. Unemployment is a very complex issue, and although counsellors will in all likelihood deal with it face-to-face with many clients, the roots of unemployment lie in the macro societal stratum of our political-economic structures. It seems important, therefore, to identify a few of these issues, as counsellors are inevitably confronted by clients who do not understand why they are in this predicament. Thus, one needs to be aware of the extent to which specific societal and/or job market circumstances contributed to the client's dilemma, or the client contributed to his or her own dilemma.

One way to address this topic is to present some of the many pervading myths about these macro-societal issues. Foremost is the myth that a certain percentage of persons who are unemployed are necessary in society in order for the economy to flourish. This primitive Durkheimian thinking (probably originating in the premise that a percentage of society needs to be deviant in order for social norms to be established) became, somewhere along the line, translated by a neo-classical economist (I assume), and this myth was erroneously propagated. Japan has been operating at a less than 1 per cent unemployment rate for the past decade and its economic growth has been unparalleled. Further, the direct (e.g., revenue, tax revenue lost, unemployment benefits, support payments) and indirect (health, welfare, and social) costs incurred in countries such as Canada and the United States render this myth truly absurd (Kirsh, 1983; Sherraden, 1985; US Congressional Budget Office, 1982).

The second myth is that it is an important value for all persons to be working and contributing to society and its quality of life. Somewhere in our evolution, the Protestant work ethic has become diluted in the western world and for a variety of reasons (e.g, cultural, sub-cultural, family supports, reference groups, social attitudes, mental or physical disabilities), there are a number of persons in our society who cannnot work, and/or do not want to work. Counsellors would do well in this regard to check their own values about this myth, particularly if they wish to be truly empathic with their clients or to help them with their self-determinism.

The third myth is that all persons who are unemployed are profoundly affected by this reality. This is a sweeping generalization which is also inaccurate. The literature on this issue suggests that unemployment affects persons in many different ways and it is only a small portion of those who are unemployed who are profoundly affected (Borrero, 1980; Liem and Rayman, 1982).

A final myth is that it is the person's fault if he or she is unemployed. Unfortunately, many clients "buy into" this myth and blame themselves for being unemployed (Briar, 1980; Briar, Fiedler, Sheean and Kamps, 1980). This generally results in feelings of inadequacy, overt victimization, and a misattributed sense of reality for many clients. Counsellors should assure their clients that in the majority of instances, it is really not their fault (the client's) if they are unemployed, and perpetuating such self-blaming is unhealthy to the client's well-being. It is important for counsellors to be apprised of some of these macro-societal myths which prevail about employment and the sooner they are addressed, the better.

The Consequences of Being Unemployed

There has been some empirical and theoretical justification for delineating specific and sequenced stages that a person who is unemployed goes through comparable to the stages of grief and loss in Kubler-Ross's (1969) model of death and dying (Bakke, 1934; Eisenberg and Lazarsfeld, 1935; Harrison, 1976; Powell and Driscoll, 1973; Zawadski and Lazarsfeld, 1983). These stages generally include the reactions of initial shock, optimism, pessimism, and then fatalism (Tiggeman and Winefield, 1984). It appears that it is the last stage which is associated with the more exacerbating and visible psychological and emotional effects of self-blame, loss of self-esteem, depression, and "learned helplessness" (Seligman, 1975), apparent in many persons who are chronically unemployed (Abrahamson, Seligman and Teasdale, 1978; Bakke, 1940; Buss and Redburn, 1983). Despite the efforts of some authors to diligently articulate each stage of this sequence with its consequent reaction (Borgen and Amundson, 1984; Krystal, Moran-Sackett, Thompson and Contoni, 1983), as a counsellor working in this field, I have some problems with this framework for a number of reasons.

Although this "ages and stages" thinking may make good conceptual and theoretical sense, it has limited practical application. Foremost, it is an oversimplification of the multi-faceted reactions persons have to being unemployed. Second, many clients exemplify a variety of reactions which are not stage specific (e.g., marital conflicts, alcohol and drug abuse, domestic violence, stress reactions, emotional reactions). Third, many of these stages may occur simultaneously, and it is difficult to discern readily what stage the client is experiencing at what time. Fourth, the typology cannot be applied to the vast majority of clients who cannot work, or have not worked for some time.

There are, however, a number of physiological, psychological, interpersonal, and familial consequences which have been shown to be associated with being unemployed. It is important to note at this point that causal attribution to such consequences cannot be unequivocally made from findings presented in the literature, but such consequences do appear with a degree of frequency among persons who are unemployed. Further, counsellors should be mindful that many variables (such as age, sex, education, culture, financial status, marital status, health status, occupational status, attitudes toward work and unemployment, and the nature of the occupation generally) confound and temper such findings. Also the majority of studies cited in this context involve the direct effects of unemployment on persons who were previously employed, and thus cannot be readily generalized to those persons who are chronically unemployed and who have never been employed.

The literature reveals, from a physiological perspective, that there are a variety of somatic stress-related health illnesses which are associated with being unemployed. These include: chest pains, shortness of breath, headaches, dizziness, dry mouth, fatigue, eczema, and an inability to sleep (Krystal, Moran-Sackett, Thompson and Contini, 1983; Lindeman, 1944; Shilonsky, Pren and Rose, 1937). Further, two well-known clinical studies with more rigorous methodologies have shown the direct effects of unemployment on blood pressure levels and blood serum cholesterol (generally associated with heart disease). Specifically, Kasl and Cobb (1970) used a longitudinal design with two control groups and two experimental groups, and studied the blood pressure changes and stress adjustment of men during the time of anticipated job loss, actual job loss, and re-employment. These authors found statistically significant elevations of blood pressure and pulse rates in men anticipating job loss. Further, men whose blood pressure remained high longer experienced more severe unemployment. Subsequently, Gore (1978) reported an increased propensity for illness and elevated blood serum cholesterol levels among men who had lost their jobs. One interpretation of all of these physiological findings is that there are both primary and secondary reactions to unemployment which are mainly manifested through the stress response cycle. The extent to which they are apparent, visible, or detrimental to the long and short term health of the person is less well known.

Psychologically, it has been determined that unemployment deals a heavy blow to many of its victims. Further, it appears that the supports a person has during unemployment – namely financial, familial, friends or social – serve as a buffer to many of the adverse psychological affects (Dean and Lin, 1977; Gore, 1978). Most often cited in the literature are feelings of loss, guilt, poor self-esteem, grief reactions, a loss of personal identity, worry and uncertainty about the future, a loss of purpose, and acute and chronic depression (Hartley, 1980; Hill, 1978; Komarovsky, 1940; Krystal *et al.*, 1983; Swinburne, 1980a). Further, Briar (1978) and Briar *et al.*, (1980) spent a good deal of time defining the "blaming syndrome" which victimizes many persons who are unemployed, and usually intertwines itself with lowered self-esteem and eventually self-degradation and then depression. Since there are few resources available to those who are unemployed (i.e., settings they can go to for counselling), many of these psychological consequences become exacerbated over time.

Interpersonally, the literature suggests that relationship skills may be affected by being unemployed. Social support is frequently and significantly identified as important in ameliorating the stressful effects of being unemployed (Keefe, 1984). In regard to the former, persons who are unemployed and who usually feel bad about their situation often feel insecure about their relationship skills (Madonia, 1983). Many may choose to withdraw from relationships and tend to alienate themselves and their families, friends, acquaintances, or social contacts (Ginzburg, 1943). Quite frankly, it really is not much fun interacting with persons who were colleagues or co-workers, or others who are constant reminders of the inadequacy of a person's station in life. Further, prolonged unemployment often results in the loss of friends. Some old ones are lost, yet sometimes new friends are found (Borrero, 1980). For example,

Briar (1978) in her study of the effects of long-term unemployment on men and women, found that while they did spend more time alone, since being unemployed, they found new friends who were also unemployed.

The role that social supports play in determining how unemployment affects individuals should not be underestimated. Certainly, the effects of unemployment stressors have been shown to be greater for persons who have low perceived levels of social support (Cobb, 1976). Further, the absence of social supports or social networks is in itself a stress for many persons (Aneshensel and Stone, 1982; Gottlieb, 1983). Keefe (1984) stated that whether social supports prevent negative affective responses to unemployment or whether social support is, itself, prevented by such responses is not a settled question (p. 265). Further, if there is a reciprocal nature to social support and its interpersonal dynamics, as Froland *et al.*, (1979) suggest, it would appear that persons with characteristically negative affective responses to stress may in turn, further diminish or inhibit supportive responses from others (Keefe, 1984). The point is that social support seems to be a key variable in understanding the interpersonal adjustment of persons who are unemployed.

Unemployment generally affects family dynamics and functioning in three ways – financial, upset of family homeostasis and the precipitation of role conflict. In regard to the former, the financial stresses and strains of unemployment for a family may be devastating, particularly for those families in which the major breadwinner becomes unemployed, and/or in those families who have incurred significant debts and have bills to pay. Despite the fact that paid work is essential for psychological survival for many persons, when deprived of an income for a length of time, families are often forced to accept support payments (unemployment insurance, welfare, etc.) or to survive on the savings or generosity of others (Kirsh, 1983). It is no secret that support payments are generally inadequate for even modest levels of survival, and as a result, over time, many persons who are unemployed or their families become victims of poverty. A counsellor should not waste much time in engaging the client in financial management skills in such cases, as it usually serves to make the situation worse (i.e., cutting coupons from the newspaper to save a few cents on an item is an acceptable premise, providing you have some cents to save). Financial problems may become worse through the way in which such persons are forced to economize (Briar *et al.*, 1980)!

Since the family is a system in the classic sense of the word, the ripple or spin-off effects of unemployment generally take their toll on many family members. Having the person who is unemployed around the house for greater periods of time than normal may upset family functioning. Borrero (1980) suggests that a common reaction of individuals who are unemployed is the feeling of "going nuts or crazy" when not working. When the person who is unemployed sees the clock go round and he or she has nothing to show for it, everyone in the household is affected (Ginzberg, 1943). Further, dysfunctional communication patterns, contagious anxiety among family members, disruption of routines and activities, intimacy problems, family stability, and family relationships with other family members are more likely to be adversely rather than positively affected.

With regard to family role relationships, changes in roles often result as a consequence of unemployment. Early studies of the effects of the depression on families (Bakke, 1935; Ginzberg, 1943), up until more recent research (Briar, 1978; Komarovsky, 1971), have established that when the husband was the main breadwinner and then became unemployed, it was difficult for him to adjust to issues of status, prestige, and authority in the family. In this context, many men feel a distinct blow to their esteemed role as 'provider' when they can no longer fulfil this function for the family. In turn, this affects their feelings of humility, inadequacy, and self-esteem. This reality, in turn, causes greater stress for the wives and children of these families. This role conflict is particularly apparent when cultural mores or values reinforce a male dominated household. The effects of unemployment on children have been less well studied. However, there is some limited evidence to suggest that such children are affected in terms of lower school grades (Hall, 1931), increased encounters with the law, and more frequent conflicts with their parents (Borrero, 1980). In short, it is safe to say that the previously noted familial problems usually affect the children in the family system in a negative way and this effect varies directly with the age of the child, the number of parents and children in the household, the family's capacity to adapt and cope, the family supports, and the length of time the family has been without an income.

There have been a number of other studies which have linked a variety of factors to unemployment. They include such variables as wife abuse, child abuse, crime and delinquency, alcohol and drug abuse, sexual dysfunctioning, mental illness, suicide and suicide ideation. These are the same types of global sociological investigations that link all of these attributes to lower social class groups, certain minority groups, certain geographic and urban areas, etc. I do not put much stock in such shotgun empiricism where anything and everything is causally linked to one factor such as being unemployed. Coupled with this, is the concern that these studies tend to lack methodological rigour and common sense (a notable exception to this methodological point includes the work of Brenner, 1973, 1976, 1979).

Data have been presented indicating that certain negative consequences do, as a rule, accrue as a result of being unemployed. There are, however, some instances in which families have achieved some positive results from this potentially traumatic event. Examples include learning to manage finances more positively (in both areas of saving and spending); learning to cope, adapt, and communicate more effectively; learning to love and support one another in more meaningful ways; developing a better appreciation for the realities of work; re-training and re-locating for a better and/or more career oriented job; making new friends; and developing new social supports.

THE CLIENT - IN - CONTEXT

Prior to outlining implications for practice, it is important for counsellors to assess the client-in-context, that is, to appraise carefully the client's situation relative to unemployment. This assessment goes further than the age-old approach of 'taking the client where she or he is at' and moves toward asking why she or he is in this situation. This strategy has basically two elements to it:

1. A disability assessment;
2. A nature of work assessment.

When both are conducted, a counsellor is in a more favourable position to assess the contextual issues surrounding the client's unemployment situation and to assist the person appropriately.

Disability Assessment

The nature of a disability is often an important determinant for effecting any sort of rehabilitation counselling. As a result, counsellors should be thorough in assessing the nature of a disability, if there is one, in order to determine whether such a disability precludes the client's ability to work. Although this discussion will focus on a primary disability area, one must not be naive about the extent to which singular disabilities are multi-faceted; result from many psycho-social dynamics; and affect other aspects of the physical, psychological, emotional, and spiritual aspects of a person. Also, one should be reminded of how family and social supports, finances, access to jobs, and the job market itself prevent or enhance any disability in this regard.

Physical Disabilities. Physical disabilities are many and varied, and at one level should be assessed on the basis of whether they are long-term and chronic, or whether they are short-term and acute. More importantly, they should be assessed on the basis of whether or not they are manageable for the client. In this regard, the same disability, such as deafness, may be manageable for some clients and not for others. After a manageability assessment of the disability, the counsellor should then determine the client's motivation and readiness for work, and the extent to which such a disability precludes, curtails, or enhances the client's capacity for work. Indeed, it is important to assess thoroughly both motivation and capacity, and to ensure their degree of congruence, as clients generally have very different perceptions about what they want to do, and what they can and cannot do. In this context it is often helpful to network with other persons who have similar disabilities and are working, and encourage a site visit with the client in order to have a more realistic sense of how the disability has affected the capacity for work. Counsellors should also note that even after such an assessment, which should include a performance and vocational assessment appraisal, there is no guarantee that the job market itself will have a job suited to the needs or abilities of the client. This is a constant and particularly frustrating reality which continually confronts counsellors and clients working in this field.

Mental Disabilities. Although an oversimplification of mental disabilities, it may be useful to divide these into:

1. Developmental disabilities;
2. Chronic mental illness (e.g., psychoticism, chronic schizophrenia, manic depression, autism, incongruous ideation and behaviour, conceptual or perceptual dysfunctioning [severe disturbances of speech, memory, orientation, or hallucinations], chronic anxiety);
3. Less chronic mental illness (e.g., episodic schizophrenia, acute paranoid ideation, acute depression, acute anxiety, unusual thought content, less severe disorientation)
4. Anxiety reactions (e.g., somatic concerns, emotional withdrawal, guilt feelings, tension, hostility, uncooperativeness, excitement, grandiosity, depressive moods).

These categories, although often overlapping, seem appropriate for at least discerning initially the nature of the mental disability at first blush. Counsellors who are confronted by clients with mental disabilities require:

1. An assessment of the nature of the disability;
2. A mental (psychometric) and mental and physical assessment;
3. A medication appraisal;
4. A vocational appraisal;
5. A social and familial support assessment;
6. A motivation/capacity for work appraisal.

Rehabilitation counsellors should only attempt to do the last two and should rely on trained professionals in the health, mental health or social service systems to furnish the other diagnoses and interpretations. It is important for counsellors to acknowledge the clinical labels that such clients have, but not allow such labels to reduce the client's employment capacity. I have heard numerous anecdotes from friends, family members, and employers who were shocked and surprised at the capacity of a person with a 'profound' [their word] mental handicap to go to work, hold a job, and perform certain tasks that were initially perceived to be beyond the client's capacity.

Emotional Disabilities/Character Disorders. Emotional disabilities or character disorders are either (a) chronic or acute disturbances which are overt, or (b) chronic or acute disturbances which are masked or undetected. The former overt disturbances are easier to discern or detect and, in many cases, are attributable to psycho-social problems, family dysfunctioning, or other physical or mental disabilities (such as those previously noted). The latter masked disturbances include the inability to get along with anyone; a passive resentment of authority; a dislike of routinization or compliance; being somewhat off-centred but still able to function at many levels; a blunted affect; a negative outlook on life; narcissism; pathological or compulsive manifestations of lying, stealing, cheating, alcohol or drug abuse; obsessions with sexuality, money, and generally taking advantage of the system.

These disabilities or disorders are often masked and unless they are formally acknowledged by the client and a professional, are very difficult to assess or pinpoint accurately. They sometimes surface when they develop into more pathological behaviours (e.g., police intervention for drunkenness, public sexual deviancy, being caught cheating or stealing, or being unable to hold a job for any length of time). Counsellors can do little more than disregard their presence until the issue becomes publicly scrutinized.

With regard to those previously acknowledged disabilities or overt disorders, counsellors need to carefully appraise whether such disabilities/disorders affect the client's willingness and capacity to work. Again, relying on professionals in the health, mental health and social service systems seems necessary for rendering such assessments.

The point of discussing these disability assessments is that, oftentimes, counsellors engage the client in some aspect of rehabilitation or vocational counselling without thoroughly coming to grips with the nature of the disability. Thus, inadvertently, they may help clients become re-employed only to have their employment setting or themselves at a later stage break down. It is worth the time to conduct a disability assessment as this is the first step toward any subsequent successful intervention. If no disability is apparent, counsellors then need to move on to the next stage of assessing the client in context, that is, determining the nature of work and unemployment with the client.

An Assessment of the Nature of Work and Unemployment

The nature and meaning of work and unemployment is very different for different people. One's experiences with work and unemployment, coupled with cultural values, support systems, and the role work plays in one's life, shape how one perceives and responds to work and unemployment (Hill, 1983; Yelin, 1986). Given how we have evolved in the western world in terms of our economies, technological advances, population growth, and the very real fact that unemployment is affecting a greater number of persons each year, the issue of what role work and unemployment plays in one's life is an important concern. When further explored, this issue triggers a number of perplexing questions, realities, and dilemmas which may confront counsellors who work in this field. As a result, counsellors should be appraised of them and be able to address them if confronted by their clients. Some of the more frequent issues are:

1. Why should I work at all?;
2. Why should I work in a job that is going nowhere, or doing nothing except frustrating me and causing me stress?;
3. Why should I work in a low paying job when I can make almost as much money on employment insurance or welfare (public assistance)?;
4. Why am I considered unemployed when I have raised children at home for the past 15 years and volunteered for many community service agencies?;
5. None of my friends or neighbours work – I'm considered weird if I do;
6. I'm never happier than when I'm not working;

7. There are really no jobs available for which I'm trained;
8. It is your (you the counsellor and your agency) responsibility to find me a job;
9. I can't get a job without experience – I can't get experience without a job.

This list is not exhaustive, but as one may surmise, some of these questions or issues are not easily or readily answered. A primary concern in addressing them lies in assessing the precise nature of the client's reality regarding work and unemployment, and then assisting the client in seeking employment. Indeed, the latter (helping the client in job searching) may be contingent upon the realities of the job market and job availability (which certainly can be a frustrating reality). The main goal of the counsellor is to assist the client in seeking employment. In order to facilitate this, a fairly simple matrix which may be used in both identifying the client's situation vis-a-vis work and unemployment, and then assisting the client in job searching behaviour is presented in Figure 9.1.

Figure 9.1 - Assessing the Nature of Work/Unemployment and Job Searching Behaviour

Factors Related to the Nature of Work	Job Searching Behaviour	
	Not Looking For Work ⟶	Looking for Work
1. Can't Work	⟶	
2. Doesn't Want to Work	⟶	
3. Can't Find Work	⟶	
4. Quit Work	⟶	
5. Layed Off/Fired	⟶	
6. Job Relocation/ Retraining	⟶	

As indicated in Figure 9.1, the counsellor may use this matrix first to pinpoint the client's work or unemployment situation, and then to develop an intervention strategy aimed at facilitating job seeking behaviour. The inherent bias of this approach is that it implies that all clients, regardless of their work or unemployment situation, should be able to evolve to the looking for work category, that is, become involved in looking for work. It also implies that if a client is looking for work, the activity is meaningful and not redundant or appeasing some other need (e.g., unemployment insurance requirements, the client's family, the counsellor, the client him or herself). In other words, it becomes incumbent upon the counsellor to ensure that the job seeking behaviour is a meaningful activity and that it falls within the goals and needs of the client. Although these biases tend to cast this issue in an optimistic direction (i.e., by assuming that all clients wish help in finding employment), I have used this matrix interactively with clients and have had success with it (Holosko, 1987). Further, it helps in assessing the nature and meaning of work or unemployment for the client, and in setting up concrete goals to facilitate appropriate job seeking behaviour. The importance of job seeking behaviour as an integral component of counselling those who are unemployed has been well established in the literature (AuClair, 1979; Nichols, 1979; Sheppard and Belitsk, 1968; Swinburne, 1980b). Finally the whole issue of job seeking implies a knowledge of vocational counselling and the job market, which to some extent requires additional knowledge and skills for which counsellors are not normally trained. A few recommended readings include: Leibowitz and Lea, 1986; Lunneborg, 1983; Roessler, 1986; Rubin and Matkin, 1984; Slaney and Russell, 1987.

IMPLICATIONS FOR PRACTICE

Indeed, given the fact that a good number of persons who are unemployed show up on the caseloads of workers in health or social service agencies (BarGal and Shamir, 1985), not to mention newer areas of practice such as employee assistance programmes (Berenbeim, 1986; Holosko and Feit, 1988), practitioners must deal with this reality in their professional practice more so than they have at any other time in their history. Further, there is a convincing body of literature suggesting that short-term crisis-oriented approaches which typify interventions for people who are unemployed are unsuitable for clients who are chronically unemployed for long periods of time (Macarov, 1988; Sherraden, 1985).

Although an argument could be made for practitioners to intervene at policy-making levels of government or human service organizations, and to lobby for changes in macro policies (e.g., income maintenance, job creation, welfare disincentive programmes) which would certainly help the plight of many persons who are unemployed, the reality is that many professions have not had access to such avenues, nor do they know how to influence them effectively. Despite the idealistic rhetoric of some authors in this regard (see Macarov, 1988, for a good example of this), the reality facing front-line practitioners is that growing numbers of persons who are unemployed are swelling their caseloads each day, and even if intervention is deemed as reactive or 'stop-gap' in its approach, we still have an ethical and professional responsibility to serve the needs of these clients. This poses a very real challenge for practitioners which is certainly a difficult, but not insurmountable, reality.

The assumptions which have been put forward in this chapter lay the foundation for some practical suggestions. First the assumptions can be summarized as follows:

1. Unemployment is a complex and multi-faceted social problem that is not well understood or even close to being resolved;
2. Unemployment is growing at an alarming rate in our society and its roots lie in the macro socio-economic and political structures;
3. Although many persons are affected by unemployment, a few of these are usually profoundly affected in an adverse way;
4. There are a variety of usually negative consequences which accrue for persons who are unemployed. These are primarily stress-related reactions (physiological, psychological, emotional, and interpersonal). Social support seems to be a salient factor in how persons are affected by unemployment;
5. Very little is known about the effects of long-term or chronic

unemployment, or about persons who have never worked.
6. A counsellor requires an understanding of the client in context which includes:
   (a) a disability assessment, and;
   (b) an assessment of the nature and meaning of work and unemployment for the client;
7. Despite some literature and findings to the contrary, counsellors should (after an assessment) actively assist clients in job searching. This implies some vocational counselling knowledge and knowledge of the existing job market;
8. Little is known about how counsellors may support clients who were previously unemployed and then became employed (i.e., how to help maintain these persons in employment).

Specific Recommendations for the Practitioner

1. Clarify values – Social workers and counsellors working in this field need to come to grips with their own values, perceptions, or stereotypes about work and unemployment. Clients respond to warmth, genuineness, and empathy and quickly notice counsellors who do not project such emotions. This is not as easy as it seems, and there are many instances in which counsellors may undermine a therapeutic relationship by inadvertently lacking this sensitivity. For example, how would an individual who values work assist a client to safeguard his or her self-determinism if the person did not wish to work?

2. Avoid stigmatization – During the therapeutic relationship, it is important not to perpetuate the stigmatization of being unemployed. Such stigmatization may lead to undue stress, victimization, and self-blaming. Reminding a client (consciously or otherwise) of his or her situation does nothing to enhance a counsellor's ability to help the client.

3. Attend to the client's needs – Two levels of needs will immediately confront the counsellor working with this group of persons. One is mental/emotional health needs; the other is employment needs. Often, these needs become

enmeshed and need to be untied. The more prominent need should be prioritized in terms of attention and intervention.

4. Assess the client-in-context – As noted earlier, a disability assessment and an assessment of the nature of work and unemployment are integral to helping the client in a meaningful therapeutic context. This implies asking and confronting the 'why' question, in order to proceed to an intervention strategy.

5. Help the client in understanding the "big picture" – Many clients tend to overpersonalize their situations and it is important to help them understand in a retrospective and objective fashion, how their situation came to be. This is difficult during the immediate trauma of just becoming unemployed, but counsellors are encouraged to address this issue. Individuals often become unemployed because of circumstances totally beyond their control (e.g., being laid off, relocation, job retraining).

6. Build on strengths – When counselling persons who are unemployed and their families, it is important to build on their strengths. It is no secret that persons are more apt to respond favourably to this approach and there is limited evidence (cited earlier) which suggests that sometimes, through such adversity, good things may happen. For example, it may be positive to be fired from a job that is stressful and unproductive to the client's quality of life. Further, new friends, new support or new jobs in more rewarding contexts may occur as a result of being unemployed.

7. Address needs of those who are chronically unemployed – Persons who have been chronically unemployed or who have never been employed are different from those who were recently employed and became unemployed. Social workers and counsellors should be sensitive to the realities of their clients' needs in these situations and adapt their intervention strategies accordingly. The literature provides some evidence that this group is growing annually.

8. Foster job-seeking behaviour – Counsellors should assist clients with meaningful job seeking behaviours. This may entail: assisting in writing resumés; conducting mock employment interviews; assisting in job readiness skills; seeking retraining programmes; assisting the client with his/her presentation of self; liaising with employers and having a knowledge of job market realities; and, conducting performance or vocational assessments. The last two activities may involve seeking other professional supports (e.g., vocational counsellors, psychometrists, psychologists).

9. Develop support groups – There is evidence in the literature for linking clients with mutual support or self-help groups as an adjunct to one-to-one counselling. These groups seem to be effective in providing support to the client through others who are in similar situations.

10. Build leisure time support – When clients who were otherwise employed become unemployed, they often do not know how to spend their newly found leisure time. As well, clients who are unemployed for a long period of time may use their leisure time in inappropriate ways. It is important, therefore, for counsellors to assist clients in adjusting to their realities and to help them in using their leisure time in productive or constructive ways.

11. Network with communities – This is an important part of counselling persons who are unemployed, as the practitioner needs to access and network with their respective communities (i.e., both health and social services, as well as employment services and employers) in order to be effective in this regard.

12. Goal setting – Using some sort of goal directed intervention, including short and long-term goals, has proven successful. In this regard, counsellors are encouraged to set both realistic and obtainable goals and also to work with the client in setting such goals.

13. Maintain a positive attitude – Counselling such clients, in particular persons who are chronically unemployed or

persons with families and bills to pay, can sometimes prove frustrating for a counsellor. It is easy in this situation to inadvertently 'feed' the victimization syndrome of many clients particularly if they have been victimized by circumstances beyond their control. It is important to maintain wherever possible a positive attitude, tempered with realism, and to facilitate the intervention to the best of your ability.

SUMMARY

In this chapter, an overview of salient issues related to counselling people who are unemployed is presented. The emphasis of the chapter focused on selected issues relating to micro-counselling (face-to-face intervention with individuals, small groups, or families). The information presented is generic and applicable to a variety of counsellors working in this field (e.g., social workers, rehabilitation counsellors, vocational counsellors, social service counsellors). Through the information presented, I have attempted to simplify (but not oversimplify) a very complex social problem. Finally, unemployment is a very real and growing problem which confronts a number of health and social service personnel on a daily basis, and until such time that its prevalence triggers a change in our political and economic structures, our institutions, and their policies, it will continue to be exacerbated.

END NOTE

1. I wish to acknowledge the insights and supports of a good friend and colleague, Dr. Gerald Erickson, Director of the School of Social Work, Windsor, Ontario, in writing this chapter. I will dearly miss both you and your insights.

REFERENCES

Abrahamson, L.Y., Seligman, M. and Teasdale, J.D. (1978) 'Learned Helplessness in Humans: Critique and Reformulation', *Journal of Abnormal Psychology, 87*, 49–74.

Aneshensel, C. and Stone, J. (1982) 'Stress and Depression: A Test of the Buffering Model of Social Support', *Archives of General Psychology, 39*, December, 1392–1396.

AuClair, P.A. (1979) 'Employment Search Decisions Among AFDC Recipients', *Social Work Research and Abstracts, 15*, 18–26.

Bakke, E.W. (1934) *The Unemployed Man*, Nesbitt Publishers, London.

Bakke, E.W. (1940) *Citizens Without Work: A Study of the Effects of Unemployment Upon the Workers, Social Relations and Practices*, Yale University Press, New Haven.

BarGal, D. and Shamir, B. (1985) 'Personnel Directors' and Welfare Officers' View of Occupations: Welfares' Role', *Social Work Papers, 19*, 56–64.

Beales, H.L., and Lambert, R.S. (1934) *Memoirs of the Unemployed*, Gollancz Publishers, London

Berenbeim, R.E. (1986) *Company Programs to Ease the Impact of Shutdowns*, The Conference Board Inc., New York.

Beveridge, W.H. (1930) *Unemployment: A Problem of Industry*, George Allen and Unwin, London.

Borgen, W.A., and Amundson, N.E. (1984) *The Experience of Unemployment*, Nelson Publishing, Scarborough, ON.

Borrero, M. (1980) 'Psychological and Emotional Impact of Unemployment', *Journal of Sociology and Social Welfare ,7*, 916–934.

Brenner, M.H. (1973) *Mental Illness and the Economy*, Harvard University Press, Cambridge, MA.

Brenner, M.H. (1976) *Estimating the Social Costs of a National Economic Policy: Implications for Mental and Physical Health and Criminal Violence*. Report prepared for the Joint Economic Committee of Congress, US Government Printing Office, Washington.

Brenner, M.H. (1979) 'Influence of the Social Environment on Psychopathology: The Historic Perspective', in J.E. Barrett (ed), *Stress and Mental Disorder*, Raven Press, New York.

Briar, K.H. (1978) *The Effect of Long-Term Unemployment on Workers and Their Families*, R and E Research Associates, San Francisco.

Briar, K.H. (1980) 'Helping the Unemployed Client', *Journal of Sociology and Social Welfare ,7*, 895–906.

Briar, K.H., Fiedler, D., Sheean, C. and Kamps, P. (1980) 'The Impact of Unemployment on Young, Middle-aged and Aged Workers', *Journal of Sociology and Social Welfare*, 7, 907–915.

Buss, T.F., and Redburn, F.S. (1983) *Mass Unemployment*, Sage Publishing, Beverly Hills.

Cobb, S. (1976) 'Social Support as a Moderator of Life Stress', *Psychosomatic Medicine*, 38, 300–314.

Dean, A., and Lin, N. (1977) 'The Stress Buffering Role of Social Support: Problems and Prospects for System Investigation', *Journal of Nervous and Mental Disorders*, 165, December, 403–417.

Eisenberg, P. and Lazarsfeld, P. (1935) 'The Psychological Effects of Unemployment', *Psychological Bulletin* , 35, June, 378.

Froland, C., Brodsy, G., Olson, M. and Stewart, L. (1979) 'Social Support and Social Adjustment: Implications for Mental Health Professionals,' *Community Mental Health Journal*, 15, 82–93.

Ginzberg, E. (1943) *The Unemployed*, Harper, New York.

Gore, S. (1978) 'The Effect of Social Support in Moderating the Health Consequences of Unemployment,' *Journal of Health and Social Behaviour*, 9, June, 157–165.

Gottlieb, B.H. (1983) *Social Support Strategies: Guidelines for Mental Health Practice*, Sage Publications, Beverly Hills.

Hall, H. (1931) *Case Studies of Unemployment*, University of Pennsylvania Press, Philadelphia.

Harrison, R. (1976) 'The Demoralizing Experience of Prolonged Unemployment', *Department of Employment Gazette*, 84, 339-348.

Hartley, J. (1980) 'The Impact of Unemployment Upon the Self-esteem of Managers', *Journal of Occupational Psychology*, 53, 147–155.

Haveman, R.H., and Wolfe, B. (1984) 'The Decline in the Male Labor Force Participation: Comment', *Journal of Political Economics*, 92(3), 532–541.

Hill, J.M. (1978) *The Social and Psychological Impact of Unemployment: A Pilot Study*, Tavistock Institute of Human Relations, London.

Hill, R. (1983) *The Meaning of Work and the Reality of Unemployment*, The Community Services Council of Newfoundland and Labrador, St. John's Newfoundland.

Holosko, M.J. (1987) 'A Model for Evaluating Rehabilitation Programs: The Case Example of the St. John's Job Generation Project', in R.I. Brown (ed), *Special Edition in Vocational*

Counselling in Rehabilitation – NATCON 14, Minister of Supply and Services Canada, Ottawa.

Holosko, M.J. and Feit, M.D. (1988) *Evaluation of Employee Assistance Programs*, Haworth Press Inc., New York.

Johnson, G.E. (1983) 'Potentials of Labour Market Policy: A View from the Eighties', *Industrial Relations*, 22(2), 283–297.

Kasl, S., and Cobb, S. (1970) 'Blood Pressure Change in Men Undergoing Job Loss: A Preliminary Report', *Psychosomatic Medicine*, 32(1), 19–38.

Keefe, T. (1984) 'The Stresses of Unemployment', *Social Work*, 29(3), 264–259.

Kirsh, S. (1983) 'Cry and You Cry Alone: What Can We Do Together?', in S. Kirsh *Unemployment: Its Impact on Body and Soul*, Canadian Mental Health Association, 85–95.

Komarovsky, M. (1940) *The Unemployed Man and His Family*, Dryden Press, New York.

Komarovsky, M. (1971) *The Unemployed Man and His Family: The Effects of Unemployment Upon the Status of the Man in Fifty-Nine Families*, Octagon Books, New York.

Krafchik, M. (1985) 'Unemployment and Vagrancy in the 1930s: Deterence, Rehabilitation and the Depression', *Journal of Social Policy*, 12(2) 195–214.

Krystal, E., Moran-Sackett, M., Thompson, S. and Contoni, L. (1983) 'Serving the Unemployed', *The Journal of Contemporary Social Work*, 64(2), 67-76.

Kubler-Ross, E. (1969) *On Death and Dying*, MacMillan, New York.

Leibowitz, Z.B., and Lea, H.D. (eds), (1986) *Adult Career Development Concepts, Issues, Practices*, National Career Development Association.

Liem, R. and Rayman, P. (1982). 'Health and Social Costs of Unemployment', *American Psychology*, 37(10), 1116–1123.

Lindeman, E. (1944) 'Symptomology and Management of Acute Grief', *American Journal of Psychiatry*, 101, 141–148.

Lunneborg, P. (1983) 'Career Counselling Techniques', in N.B. Walsh and S.H. Osipow (eds), *Handbook of Vocational Psychology – Volume 2 – Applications*, 41–77, Lawrence Erlbaum Associates Inc., New Jersey.

Macarov, D. (1988) 'Re-evaluation of Unemployment', *Social Work*, 33(1), 23–27.

Madonia, J. (1983) 'The Trauma of Unemployment and its Consequences', *Social Casework*, 64(2), 482–488.

Nichols, A.C. (1979) 'Why Welfare Mothers Work: Implications for Employment and Training Service', *Social Services Review*, 53, 378–391.

O'Brien, G.E. (1985) 'Distortion in Unemployment Research: The Early Studies on Baake and their Implications for Current Research on Employment and Unemployment', *Human Relations*, 38(9), 877–894.

Perry, G.L. (1972) 'Unemployment Flows in the U.S. Labour Market', in *Brookings Papers on Economic Activity* , 245-278, Brookings Institute.

Powell, D. and Driscoll, P. (1973) 'Middle Class Professionals Face Unemployment', *Society, 10*, 18–26.

Reigle, D.W. (1982) 'The Psychological and Social Effects of Unemployment,' *American Psychology*, 37(18), 1113–1115.

Roessler, R.T. (1986) 'Training for Vocational Coping: A Method for Establishing Work Establishment Skills', *Rehabilitation Counseling Bulletin*, 29(4), 258–265.

Rubin, S.E. and Matkin, R.E. (1984) 'Roles and Functions of Certified Rehabilitation Counselors', *Rehabilitation Counseling Bulletin*, 27(4), 199–224.

Seligman, M.E. (1975) *Helplessness*, W.H. Freeman, San Francisco.

Sheppard, H.L. and Belitsk, A.M. (1968) 'Promoting Job Finding Success for the Unemployed', in *The W.E. Upjohn Institute for Employment Research Papers*, Kalamazoo, Michigan.

Sherraden, M. (1985) 'Chronic Unemployment: A Social Work Perspective', *Social Work, Sept-Oct*, 403–408.

Shilonsky, H., Pren, P. and Rose, M. (1937) 'Clinical Observations on the Reactions of a Group of Transients to Unemployment', *Journal of Social Psychology, 8*, 81–82.

Slaney, R.B. and Russell, J.E. (1987) 'Perspectives on Vocational Behavior, 1986: A Review', *Journal of Vocational Behavior, 31*, 111–173.

Swinburne, P. (1980a) 'The Psychological Impact of Unemployment on Managers and Professional Staff', *Journal of Occupational Psychology, 53*, 48–60.

Swinburne, P. (1980b) 'Unemployment in 1980 – The Experience of Managers and Professional Staff', *Employee Relations, 3*(3), 48–60.

Tiggeman, M. and Winefield, A.M. (1984) 'The Effects of Unemployment on the Mood, Self-esteem, Locus of Control and Depressive Affect of School Leavers', *Journal of Occupational Psychology, 57*, 33–42.

USA (1982) *'The Economic and Budget Outlook: An update,'* US Congressional Budget Office Papers, US Government Printing Office, Washington, D.C.

Yelin, E. (1986) 'The Myth of Malingering: Why Individuals Withdraw from Work in the Presence of Illness', *The Milbank Quarterly*, 64(4),622–649.

Zawadski, B. and Lazarsfeld, P. (1983) 'The Psychological Consequences of Unemployment', *Journal of Social Psychology*, 6(2), 224–251.

Chapter Ten

COUNSELLING PERSONS WHO ARE DEAF

Gunnel Backenroth

INTRODUCTION

It is perhaps especially within Swedish psychology that a polarization has arisen between diagnosis and treatment. Both diagnosis and treatment were responses to manifest needs in society, and society consequently provided the necessary resources for them. At present there are new needs in society which psychologists and researchers should be prepared to meet, using preventive measures which aim to optimize the individual's developmental potential and create the prerequisites for a better life for various groups of persons with disabilities. The present chapter, to a large extent, refers to research and practice in the area of preventive psychology. The references to the author's research concern studies carried out in conjunction with the Swedish National Association for the Deaf and financed by the Delegation for Social Research (DSF) and the Allmanna Arvsfonden (the Inheritance Foundation).

By systematically collecting and reviewing experience and knowledge, we increase not only our "cultural competence" in relevant areas but also our understanding of various aspects of individual development and of conditions in society. Using our research results and experience as a baseline, we can influence the attitudes of society toward people with handicaps and their families, utilize resources in the best manner possible, and hopefully improve the living conditions of persons who have handicaps and their families. Handicapping conditions represent one of the most important areas in which psychology assumes a central role (Fenderson, 1984). Nevertheless, while psychological competence is certainly important, research in the field of handicap requires interdisciplinary and professional competence.

If one studies international developments in the field of deafness, three developmental trends can be discerned. First, researchers are ceasing to compare people who are deaf with those with unimpaired hearing and have discontinued regarding deafness as a deviation from normal hearing status. Rather, the emphasis is now placed on capacity and capabilities (Ahlgren, 1978; Backenroth, 1987a; Backenroth and Hanson, 1987; Basilier, 1964, 1973; Bergman, 1982; Norden, 1975, 1981; Preisler, 1983; Remvig, 1969) and comparative studies now concern comparison within the deaf population (Levine, 1976).

Second, researchers have begun to recognize that the field of deafness represents an heterogeneous group of people rather than a homogeneous group or a single deaf personality. However, there are still only a few documented studies that characterize this population as showing a high degree of heterogeneity (Backenroth and Hanson, 1986, 1987; Levine, 1976). In earlier personality studies people with deafness usually fared badly when compared to those with unimpaired hearing. The literature describes people who are deaf as conforming, suspicious, poorly adapted to reality, inclined to authoritarianism (Axelsson and Crafoord, 1975), immature, rigid (Axelsson and Crafoord, 1975; Levine, 1976), misfits and dependents (Levine, 1976), isolated and incapable of establishing close relations (Jongkees, 1983; Pyke and Littman, 1982), introverted (Jongkees, 1983), and depressive (Mahapatra, 1974).

Third, the researcher's role in the field of deafness has changed. The researcher instead of being primarily an observer, has become a more active participant in the research process (Levine, 1976). Nowadays, the researcher may even take part in the "treatment" as therapist (see Backenroth, 1983; Backenroth and Hanson, 1987). Goldman (1976) claims that an important aspect of counselling is the counsellor's role as the most important instrument of research.

The starting point for research in Sweden during the first half of the 1970s, as in so many other countries, lay in the debate over the status of sign language which dominated the area. At the same time, the psychological aspects of deafness had been overridden by the technical, medical, and pedagogical aspects (Backenroth, 1983). Furthermore, the child with deafness had constantly been the focus of research interest (Backenroth, 1975, 1976, 1983), a development which was also becoming evident in the USA (Mindel and Vernon, 1971; Schlesinger and Meadow, 1972). Society's resources had been invested primarily in child rehabilitation, which was necessary but not sufficient.

It has gradually become more apparent that measures aimed only at the child have limited effect if the emotional needs of the parents are not adequately addressed at the same time (Mindel and Vernon, 1971). Whenever the literature in the area of handicap has focused on parents, the parents have mainly been caretakers of children (Backenroth, 1983). Furthermore, when the parents have come under study, attention has been paid primarily to the mother and her role in relation to the child with the handicap (Backenroth, 1984a).

In the present organization of hearing care in Sweden – which is currently under review – there is still a strong emphasis on pedagogical issues and the personnel associated with these aspects. There is an historical explanation for this. Previously child rehabilitation was seen as an educational problem and the emphasis was placed on structural speech therapy programmes. In more recent years, a stronger emphasis on psychological factors has been sought, both in Sweden and in other parts of the world. This is important for both parents and/or children with handicaps themselves (Backenroth, 1983; Backenroth and Hanson, 1986, 1987; Menolascino and Coleman, 1980; Vernon, 1972). The present chapter focuses on individuals who are deaf at birth or whose deafness dates from early childhood, and their parents.

BASIC VIEWPOINTS IN THE DEAF AREA

There has been considerable reliance on "experts" in the field of deafness for many years. Medical, pedagogical and technical personnel have predominated within this area. The basic policy has not been to "develop competence" amongst those who are deaf but rather to concentrate on what the individuals lack in relation to those with hearing. An examination of both research and practice supports this assertion.

An alternative approach arises from a psychodynamic viewpoint (Backenroth, 1978, 1983) combined with humanistic ideas (Backenroth, 1989; Backenroth and Hanson, 1986;

Goldstein, 1986; Raubolt, 1985) and these can form a useful frame of reference for a different "professional approach" in this field. Humanistic psychology, however, still has insufficient influence on the attitudes of professionals. It is still not unusual for "experts", instead of asking what persons who are deaf actually want, to tell them what is best for them. The importance of respecting the wishes and concerns of the consumers – people with deafness and their families – when measures are proposed, cannot be sufficiently emphasized. It is necessary, if not to say fruitful, to establish close and honest relationships between people who are deaf and their families and ourselves, the professionals. The person who is deaf must always play the key role in situations that concern him or her since it is his or her own future and life situation that is at stake. This standpoint is supported by Vernon (1970, 1975) and Steele (1976).

The family is the central concept in many rehabilitation programmes. But is parent support sufficient to give the child with deafness positive opportunities for development? Is a single working model a sufficient basis from which to work? And is it possible to solve the psychosocial problems of adults who were deaf as children by means of counselling or therapy? Perhaps we need to work in parallel on several different levels. Furthermore, are we sufficiently prepared as professionals to meet the needs of the person with deafness and those of his or her family? What possibilities exist? In practice a fertile approach has been to use a model which allows for measures on several different levels at the same time: intrapsychic, interpersonal and structural. The working model presented in Backenroth and Hanson (1986) has been developed from a counselling model described by Morrill, Oetting, and Hurst (1974) and Drapela (1983). It is apparent that counsellors work frequently within a limited segment of this model. The tendency seems to be to focus on the individual and the family (target) and on corrective measures (purpose). The method itself usually comprises direct support in the form of counselling or information (Backenroth and Borgen, 1987).

IMPORTANCE OF THE SOCIAL NETWORK

The social network is important for the individual's psychic and physical well-being and health. We cannot thrive without family, friends, relations, neighbours, work colleagues or bosses who care about us. During the last decade an interest has arisen, particularly in epidemiological research, in the association between social relations and health (Caplan, 1981; Cassel, 1974; Gottlieb, 1985; Östergren, 1984; Svedhem *et al.*, 1985). Cassel (1974) has shown that changes in the social environment are reflected in the general level of resistance to illness. He strongly stresses that an absence of social feedback is a predominant cause of an increased susceptibility to illness. Gottlieb (1985) argues that illness often follows disruptive experiences in an individual's life, such as divorce, unemployment or moving. Such changes influence the immunity levels and render the individual more liable to illness.

Social support is important as a preventive measure against illnesses arising from stress or handicap (Gottlieb, 1985). Caplan (1981) has described how social support can protect a person from the effects of discrepancies between oneself and the environment on six different functional levels. Svedhem *et al.* (1985) summarizes the conclusions that can be drawn from the literature about social networks and health as follows: "Get married, go to church, meet friends and relations, join a few societies" (p.82).

According to Östergren (1984) the concept of social support involves the individual's available social contacts. How the individual experiences this social support depends to a large extent on the social transactions which occur. Social contact can be defined as "the feedback provided via contact with similar and valued peers" (Gottlieb, 1985, p.9). Gottlieb argues that social support can be seen from three viewpoints. First, on the macro level where social support is measured in terms of social integration. Second, on the mezzo level where one measures structure and the supportive function of the network. Third, on the micro level where one examines more the quality of the relations than the quantity. Sarason, Sarason and Shearin (1986) have shown that the stability period of social support is three years. Robertson (1988), summarizing this work, proposed that social support consists of four different support resources: esteem support (emotional or expressive support), informational support (advice, appraisal support, cognitive guidance), social companionship (belongingness) and instrumental support (material resources).

The social network comprises all the people who are relevant for an individual at any point in time, and the relationships between them and the person in question

(Östergren, 1984). Robertson (1988) considers it important to point out that the social network can have destructive consequences for the individual as well as constructive ones. Another important point which is emphasized is that social support is by no means static. Interaction with a particular individual in the social network can be supportive on one occasion and conflict-laden on another.

In the following sections a presentation of the social networks of people with deafness is given from three different perspectives. The first section lays the emphasis on the child who is deaf and the primary reference group, the family ("the emotional network"). The second section focuses on the adult with deafness and his or her secondary group - peers, club mates, etc. (the social network). The third section stresses the adult with deafness in relation to society, in this case the people who work among people with deafness (the professional interpreter network). I have borrowed the terms emotional, social and professional networks from Crafoord (1987). In order to release the personal powers of development and problem solving of persons with deafness, it is important to try and influence the networks at different levels (Backenroth and Hanson, 1987).

THE PERSON WHO IS DEAF AND THE EMOTIONAL NETWORK

The primary group (i.e., the family) is of extreme importance for the individual's well-being and acts as a "buffer" against the psychological and physical consequences of stress situations (Cassel, 1976). The emotional network comprises those persons on whom the individual is emotionally dependent. For the majority of people this means the family (Craaford, 1987).

The family is the stable environment in which the child develops his or her personality. The relations between mother, father and child are important for how the child experiences others with whom he or she comes in contact. It is through the feelings shown toward the child that the child will experience him or herself as an individual. The parents play a decisive role as the child's most important environmental contact, regardless of whether the child is deaf or of normal hearing. Interaction and communication between the child and his or her parents play a critical role in the development of the child's personality and in his or her intellectual, social and cultural development.

Every year in Sweden 200 families are informed that their child is deaf or hearing impaired. In the majority of cases this leads to strong emotional reactions and for many parents results in a psychological crisis with varying degrees of chronic consequences (Backenroth, 1983). The parental role is normally associated with positive expectations and opportunities as well as enriching experiences for one's own personality. According to Meadow (1969), socialization for many parents of children with handicaps involves a transition to a role with undesired and lower status.

All parents need understanding and support in order to function better in their parental role. The parents' expectations are generally based on experiences and knowledge of the child who is without handicap. Parents of children with deafness and hearing-impairments require extra support since the role of a parent to a child that cannot hear involves new difficulties that parents of children with normal hearing never meet. Being the parent of a child who is deaf can feel "as if the parental burden has been increased by a few kilos, and one's opportunities reduced" (quote from a parent in a counselling group, see Backenroth, 1978).

The parents must teach themselves and their child to live with and accept deafness. They must adjust their expectations and their outlook to the child's somewhat different prospects, appreciate the child's difficulties in certain situations and at the same time give priority to helping the child develop his or her capabilities as well as possible. The family with a member who is deaf can be seen from a systems theory perspective (Backenroth, 1983) as an open and dynamic system in which the family members exert a mutual influence on each other and moreover where their relationship with society is also one of reciprocal influence. Not all the difficulties that parents of children with deafness experience derive from deafness, but, rather, have their roots in earlier experiences in life: experiences which have remained latent until triggered by the present situation (Backenroth, 1983). Many parents need to be able to solve their own personal problems before they can manage to involve themselves fully with their child who is deaf (Backenroth, 1978).

Direct support to the parents means indirect support to

the child. Rotter (1974) stresses that the child's most valuable assets are stable and knowledgeable parents and several researchers claim that preventive measures for parents of children with deafness are required if children are to receive optimal opportunities for development. The successful resolution of difficulties can increase the preparedness and capacity for handling future difficulties (Backenroth, 1975, 1976, 1978, 1983; Crafoord and Axelsson, 1975; Jongkees, 1983; Mindel and Vernon, 1971; Vernon, 1971). Professional parent support is necessary and a lack of adequate support at the time when deafness is diagnosed lays the ground for subsequent "family pathology" and for many of the difficulties which parents of youngsters/adults who are deaf experience (Vernon, 1971).

The character of the parents' network influences events within the family of children with handicaps. The parents' ability to give – in Robertson's terms (1988) – emotional support, appraisal support, belongingness and instrumental support affects the child both while growing up and later in life. McDowell and Gabel (1981) have found that the networks of parents of children who have handicaps are less developed than those of families whose children are without handicap. It can be said that parents of children with handicaps have a "wider meshed" network than parents of children who are not handicapped.

In the same way that children with deafness need to identify with other children/adults who are deaf, so their parents need to meet and feel affinity with other parents who are or have been in the same situation. Uncertainty in their parental role is then replaced by greater security, knowledge and impulses, as well as resources, enabling them to work actively through the handicap and fight for their child's rights in society (Backenroth, 1976, 1978).

The phenomenon of parent groups has a long history and as early as the 1880s mothers in the USA formed a group with the aim of becoming "better parents" (Auerbach, 1959, 1961). Many parent groups have now developed and constitute a dynamic learning situation based on parents' interests and needs. Parent groups have sometimes been initiated by professional group leaders, with parents as group leaders but there are also "leaderless" groups (Backenroth, 1983).

Parents of children with deafness, when finding

themselves in their new and unexpected life situation, sooner or later feel a need to meet other parents in the same situation. With other parents they can express and share mutual emotions and experiences. The feeling of "all being in the same boat" (i.e., of universality), results in group affinity, a relaxing of tension, support, and reduction of guilt feelings, and thereby forms a productive basis for being able to develop a new identity as the parent of a child with deafness. The contact with other parents also functions as a sort of "social comparison" and as reality testing in relation to the deafness itself. As a result the parents can form a frame of reference by which they are better able to judge the child's deafness and the implications of deafness in a hearing society.

Identification with a social network is one of the four important major concepts in a group counselling programme for parents of children with deafness and hearing impairments developed by Backenroth (1983). The design of this programme was inspired by Trotzer (1977) among others. The three remaining concepts involved in the programme are reality testing, "working-through" and acceptance (Backenroth, 1983, 1984a, 1984b, 1984c). The main value of this counselling programme has turned out to be, besides the working through of problems associated with the child's deafness, the establishment of a social network with other parents and reality testing in terms of an increased understanding of the handicap and the child. Parents valued the experience of identification in terms of universality, support, belonging and catharsis in the group process. Indeed parents who reported reality testing in terms of a better ability to estimate and appreciate the child's future prospects, tended to rate the benefit derived from the programme more highly (Backenroth, 1983, 1984d, 1987b).

A follow-up study showed that parents, who had reported deriving benefit from group counselling during the evaluation, also reported a benefit from counselling at the follow-up one year later. In a further follow-up 4-6 years after the completion of the counselling, identification and the creation of a contact network with parents in the same or similar circumstances were the benefits reported by the parents (Backenroth, 1984a). The follow-up studies showed that the parents' estimates of the benefits of counselling were maintained over time when the data were analyzed quantitatively (Backenroth, 1984b). The increase in the number of social contacts and the creation of a permanent social network with other parents (84%) and with deaf people (65%) constitute important results of the group counselling programme (Backenroth, 1984a). Other investigations have also shown that benefits of the group can persist as permanent social relations (Feldman, 1981; Fernlund and Gustafsson, 1981).

The parents' capacity for identification, reality testing and working through concerns and situations ought to facilitate the process of acceptance of the child, his or her deafness and the consequences of the deafness. The parents' progress toward acceptance is a process requiring both time and effort. It takes time to work through all the feelings that arise, develop the necessary insights and derive the consequences from them. Moreover new problems and decisions arise continuously. Acceptance is by no means final, but rather a process that continues throughout life. This has implications for the support and counselling that society should offer the family with a member who is deaf (Backenroth, 1983, 1984c).

A so-called picture interview (see Backenroth, 1983, 1986a) has been used in counselling parents of children who are deaf to help them work through their feelings relating to deafness. The parents' responses to the picture series works projectively and can be a guide to recognizing the key problems in the family. The picture material can be regarded as both diagnostic and therapeutic in nature. The results of one study show differences between the responses of parents who had reached acceptance, and those that were still working through the situation (Backenroth, 1986a). Parents can presumably work through their personal problems using pictures and with their help change their own conceptions of the problem situation.

Support from parental organizations is extremely important during the "working-through" process. Such organizations can come in contact with parents who are practically inaccessible to hearing care centres or research projects. A Swedish report confirms this (Backenroth, 1980).

Measures aimed at building up networks for the primary group assume cooperation with hearing care and parental organizations. All concerned have a need to utilize each other's competence and experience within the area. Secure and positive parents can give the child security and the possibility of a quality life while growing up and in adulthood. But, just as it is important that the parents function together with their children, so it is also important that the emotional network – the family with a member who has deafness – functions together with the social and professional networks. A well-functioning emotional network provides the resources to handle disruptions in the social network caused by persons on whom the individual is not as emotionally dependent (Crafoord, 1987).

THE PERSON WHO IS DEAF AND THE SOCIAL NETWORK

Social networks vary. Their pervading characteristic is that their members, in varying degrees, consist of relations, neighbours, society or club friends, work colleagues, and so on. In a social network some people, but not all, have social contact or relationships with each other. One normally differentiates between informal and formal contacts, and it is the former that most closely resemble what is meant here by social network.

There is reason to assume that self reports by people with deafness about the size and characteristics of their social networks and their satisfaction with them over a long period of time are reliable (Sarason *et al.*, 1986). Another assumption is that the basis for the social network has been laid during the individual's early years and has continued to be formed during adult life. Finally, a third assumption can be made, namely that deficiencies in the social network can be related to the parents' difficulties in accepting the individual's deafness (Backenroth, 1983, 1984c).

One line of research on social networks has concentrated on the functions filled by various key people (Greenblatt, Becerra and Serafetinides, 1982). All people have a social network and it is important, from a psychological viewpoint, to see the individual in relation to the group to which he or she belongs (Svedhem *et al.*, 1985). The need for identification models and opportunities for building up the social network of persons with deafness has been stressed (Backenroth and Hanson, 1987).

Recent research results support observations that have been made over several centuries, namely that persons with deafness, broadly speaking, have the same emotional and intellectual capacities as persons with hearing. Differences in competence between people with deafness and those with hearing usually depend on differences in language and social training (Furth, 1977; Levine, 1976; Vernon, 1970). The types of emotional disturbances which occur in the hearing also exist amongst persons with deafness (Robinson, 1971).

In Sweden there are between 8,000 – 10,000 people with deafness originating in childhood. Sign language is now the natural means of communication for children who have deafness and their families. But many older people have grown up without sign language at a time when it was not officially sanctioned in the Swedish educational system. Sign language was accepted as a language and as the primary language for the population with deafness in a parliamentary decision in 1981. The fact that sign language was recognized so late has meant that persons who have deafness and who have now reached middle age, have had less favourable developmental opportunities (Backenroth and Hanson, 1986). We can, however, feel pleasure in the fact that persons with deafness have gained respect for many of the demands they have legitimately placed on "the hearing society" during the past 20 years (Backenroth, 1989).

An association for people with deafness constitutes for many persons with deafness a psychic valve and the basis for contact and belonging. But there are persons with deafness (estimated at about 10%) who for various reasons remain outside of the community of those who have deafness. Oscar Wilde is quoted as saying that there is only one thing worse than being spoken about in one's presence, and that is not being spoken about at all. There are many persons with deafness who would not share this opinion. Experience has shown that there are many who live in self-chosen isolation not wishing to become integrated into a group of persons with deafness characterized by the spreading of gossip and rumour. At times one has reason to wonder what implications this has for mental health and the possibility of belonging to the group of those with deafness.

A central concept in relation to people who are deaf and psychosocially isolated is reality testing (see Figure 10.1). The concepts of identification, reality testing and working through are included in acceptance (Backenroth, 1984c). The concepts in the model should not be seen as separate since they interact with each other (Backenroth, 1983; 1984c; Backenroth and Hanson, 1986).

The concept of reality testing includes adapting to reality. It requires that one can take realistic decisions, and realize the consequences of having deafness in a society dominated by people with hearing (Backenroth, 1986b). Furthermore, it includes an understanding of one's own capabilities and shortcomings, and the demands of others as well as social expectations and obligations. It is a resource that facilitates the individual's interaction with other people. An approach that has gradually gained ground in psychology, is the interactionist perspective (Magnusson, Duner and Zetterblom, 1975; Sigmon, 1984). According to interactionism there is a continual reciprocal action between the individual and the situations within which he or she acts (Magnusson and Endler, 1976).

Figure 10.1   A model of the relation between the main concepts in a working model in work with persons who are deaf.

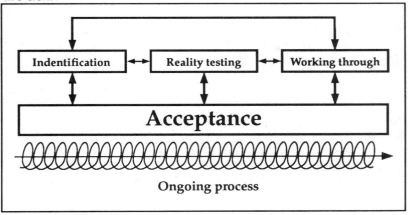

Not belonging to a group of people with deafness means isolation for a person who is deaf: it is the only group he or she has. People with hearing can choose between many different groups of hearing, but the deaf cannot do likewise. Thus the psychosocial isolation is unmercifully hard. In order to have an effect on both the internal and external factors related to isolation it is essential and productive to use a working model that can take several levels into consideration simultaneously. This is necessary if any positive changes are to be achieved in the overall situation of the person with deafness.

Psychosocial rehabilitation can take place on different levels at the same time (Backenroth and Hanson, 1986) and is both a window on and a mirror to society. Treatment aims at creating conditions for change so that the client can "fit into" society (Estroff, 1983). When we attempt to make positive changes in the social network of the person with deafness in order to liberate problem solving capacities, how often do we manage to treat those persons who reject, avoid or exclude our clients from the community of persons with deafness? Normally, there are insufficient resources for working with non-clients. Peer counselling or "discussion evenings" are aimed at this secondary group and seek to change attitudes gradually in the group of persons with deafness so that our clients meet an increased understanding for their difficulties and life situation (Backenroth and Hanson, 1986, 1987).

How well equipped is the so-called professional for working with minority groups? Sue and Zane (1987) point to the importance of reformulating the client's problems in medical terms when working with Spanish speaking groups, of avoiding interpersonal feelings and touching when dealing with Philippinos, and of being action oriented when working with black people. According to Sue (1981) and Sue and Zane (1987) society has increasingly become aware that professionals, especially in counselling and clinical psychology, have failed to meet the needs of the cultural minorities. Sue and Sue (1977) claim that minority groups who seek psychotherapeutic help are discriminated against on the grounds that psychiatric workers lack a knowledge and understanding of minority communities. Similar observations on the need for cultural competence have been made in the area of deafness (Backenroth, 1986b, 1988; Denmark, 1966; Denmark and Eldridge, 1969; Garstecki, 1982; Levine, 1976; Pyke and Littman, 1982; Schein, 1983; Sussman, 1983; Thoreson and Tully, 1971; Vernon, 1970; Williams and Sussman, 1971).

People with deafness, seen in an historical perspective, have been treated, to put it mildly, somewhat harshly. Since they are a minority group scant resources have been allocated to them. However, a lack of resources (Award, 1978) is not the only restriction. There is also insufficient preparedness to accept people with deafness (Pyke and Littman, 1982). Added to this there has been a large degree of uncertainty over the actual needs of people who are deaf. As early as the 1960s the importance of preventive measures and the need for a specialized psychiatric service for those who are deaf was stressed (Denmark, 1966; Denmark and Eldridge, 1969; Remvig, 1969). These and other needs have continued to be pointed out even into the 1980s (Schein, 1983).

How does one carry out counselling, therapy and advisory work with persons with deafness? Hoyt, Siegelman and Schlesinger (1981) have criticized the lack of guidance in the research literature as to how clinicians should conduct psychotherapy with their patients with deafness. What then is counselling in the present context? Rogers (1942) defines counselling as a series of direct contacts with the individual that aim to provide help in changing attitudes and behaviour. Patterson (1974) is of the opinion that counselling is a helping process in which the relationship itself is both necessary and important. Furthermore, he considers that counselling occurs in a non-medical setting, otherwise it is called psychotherapy. Counselling has become an increasingly applied specialty, Fitzgerald and Osipow (1986) found in one study that counsellors considered they were more engaged in psychotherapy and traditional clinical activities than in vocational counselling, academic counselling or research-focused activities.

Research into individual counselling with people with deafness (a study where one of the counsellors was deaf) has shown that the individual's need of support and the nature of the social network, vary with the occurrence of psychosocial problems. All individuals who are deaf have, albeit in varying degrees, need of help in developing their social networks working through situations and adapting to reality (Backenroth and Hanson, 1986, 1987).

Society needs to recognize the advantages of being bicultural, according to Baratz and Baratz (1970). It is important that counsellors receive professional education for example, and involve ethnic minorities: "Although many white professionals have great understanding and empathy for minorities, they can never fully appreciate the dilemmas faced by a minority member" (Sue, 1981, p.20). At the same time it is important to be aware of the inherent difficulties. Solomon (1976) for example, argues that therapists who themselves are deaf on the one hand represent a resource in therapeutic work providing they have acquired education and clinical experience, and have undergone therapy and training. On the other hand the therapist with deafness is confronted with other problems that do not arise for the hearing therapist.

THE PERSON WHO IS DEAF AND THE PROFESSIONAL INTERPRETER NETWORK

When we consider the more formal contacts in the social network of the person with deafness, we mean the professional network, since this consists of the professional helpers with whom the person, to a greater or lesser extent, has contact. In this section the emphasis is on those professionals, namely interpreters, upon whom many consumers or clients are most dependent for realizing their opportunities in society (education, employment, family recreation).

In this context cultural affiliation is both a powerful but also sometimes a subtle determinant of an individual's perceptual and cognitive world, and of his or her behavioural repertoire. Culture determines when we seek help from professional helpers and from whom we seek help. Just as our minority groups in society have a lot to teach us on the basis of their experiences so the interpreters have a great deal to teach us on the basis of their unique competence in the culture of those with deafness. Opportunities for further education in areas where they can use their expert knowledge are important for people with deafness (Backenroth, 1986b, 1987a, 1989). In this respect they are dependent on the availability of interpreters (Backenroth, 1986b, 1987a, 1989). The ultimate aim is to provide persons who are deaf with a qualified interpreter service. The situation in Sweden at present is such that it is difficult to provide the required service since the demand for interpreters far exceeds the supply. An increasing number of people with deafness continue to higher education, and moreover are to be found in positions in society which necessitate the use of interpreters for meetings, courses and conferences.

Interpretation services have changed character and the interpreter's role is rapidly changing. There are today about 300 interpreters in Sweden. This group is no longer homogeneous either in background experience, (i.e., a genuine historical connection with the community of those with deafness), or in everyday experience (Backenroth, 1986b, 1987a), and an expansion of the interpreter service is required to facilitate the consumer's self-actualization (Backenroth, 1989).

The interpreter's identity as an interpreter develops in an interaction between the interpreter and the environment within which he or she lives and works. The interpreter can easily identify with the person with deafness and his or her needs. In many situations a conflict of interests arises for the interpreter. The interpreter feels primarily for the person who is deaf and who, in certain cases, wishes the interpreter to support him or her openly. Interpreters who have parents with deafness know what their parents missed. The interpreter feels a pleasure in being able to help. This personal involvement and competence in the culture of persons with deafness can be both a resource and a burden. The interpreter unconsciously assumes the attitudes and difficulties of the person with deafness and feels a "responsibility" for ensuring that people regard the individual (and the persons with deafness in general) in a positive light. The interpreter attempts the whole time to present the person with deafness in the right way and communicate the "best" possible language (Backenroth, 1988).

The consumer of interpreter services often has an ambivalent attitude toward the interpreter. On the one hand he or she has to have an interpreter, but on the other wishes that this was not needed. Both people with deafness and with hearing can feel an unconscious irritation over their dependence on the interpreter. The interpreter is affected by the so-called "super-interpreter syndrome", living under an unhealthy demand to be perfect, and to work continually without making a single mistake (Backenroth, 1988). The interpreter can never be totally prepared for an assignment and there is only a small degree of personal control in the work itself. The interpreter has to work under physical and psychological pressure with little possibility of airing or working through one's feelings. The interpreter's work often involves making the most of impossible working conditions. It is a "risk" profession with a high risk of "burnout" (Backenroth, 1988).

Interpreters need to have opportunities to ventilate and work through these problems. There is a need for "interpreter focused personnel supervision" (Backenroth, 1988; 1989) to allow interpreters to reinforce their professional identity, gain self-confidence and regain or maintain a constructive perspective on their work – in short they need to be supported in offering an adequate professional network to people with deafness. Well-functioning interpreters, both on assignments and in cooperation with each other, are a prerequisite for a qualified interpretation service for the community of persons with deafness!

SUMMARY AND RECOMMENDATIONS

The total social network of the person with deafness can be seen as an open and dynamic system in which each link (the emotional, the social and the professional) influences the others. This system helps the individual to maintain an interactive relationship with the environment. The persons included in each link of the "chain of security" of the person with deafness have a common responsibility for the individual's psychological health. The people involved in this network also need resources and support of various kinds in order to function well in their roles linking (developmentally, emotionally, cognitively, socially and culturally) the person with deafness with his or her environment.

The most important factors for the social network of the persons with deafness are the following:

1. Positive attitudes to deafness, sign language and deaf culture;
2. Contact with other people who are deaf;
3. Parents who have contact with other parents and with the community of persons with deafness;
4. Early and continuing parental support;
5. Access to qualified interpreters;
6. Access to professionals with a mastery of sign language and intimate knowledge of the deaf culture;
7. Access to a variety of supportive resources for the person with deafness and his or her family, as well as access to

professionals working with families of persons with deafness;
8. Cooperation between emotional, social and professional networks.

To ensure optimal developmental conditions for consumers, who are deaf, preventive measures aimed at different levels are required, where attention can be paid to the creation and development of emotional, social and professional networks. The potential opportunities for the child with deafness to develop in our society depend on such conditions as the communication and interaction between parents and child and the family's as well as society's attitudes, values and possibilities. Specific recommendations for work with persons who are deaf and those in their social networks follow.

1. When a family learns that their child is deaf or hearing impaired, adequate information and support are necessary – for example individual counselling or group counselling. Many parents feel the need to solve their own personal problems and difficulties before they can engage in the activities offered by hearing care centres, nursery schools and parent organizations. Understanding, acceptance, empathy and appropriate 'timing' of interventions are necessary ingredients in a professional approach to parents. All professionals must be well informed about the parental needs. Various studies (Backenroth, 1983) show the importance and necessity of an adequate and continuing parental support programme to ensure a favourable developmental climate for children with deafness. Parents of children who have handicaps can, and often do, require specialized support during critical periods of the child's life. Thus, "parent care" should be offered as a matter of course and may be seen as a parental right as new difficulties and decisions arise. Since parents of children who are deaf comprise such a heterogeneous group with varying needs, future services must be prepared to deal with practical realities so that parents can be offered different models of support (Backenroth, 1984a). Parents' competence must be recognized so that their resources and activities can be utilized effectively in the child's rehabilitation.

2. Parallel to parental support, people with deafness also require and seek support involving counselling or psychiatric help

during different phases of life. They must be attended by personnel who have a mastery of sign language and communication. Thus, sign language education must be increased and offered at a qualitatively higher level than at present to many groups. These include parents, 'day care mothers', personnel in day care centres, nursery schools, special schools, hospitals, employers and employees in work units where people with deafness work, staff in outpatient psychiatric clinics, and personnel in care units for the elderly.

3. Personnel working with the family of persons with deafness need to work through their own attitudes and their professional approach of those who are deaf on an on-going basis. Overprotection needs to be minimized in favour of increased support which champions the development of self-confidence, competence, decision-making skills (particularly those relating to educational/professional aspirations and employment), responsibility, realistic attitudes and increased participation in society.

4. The social environment of family, friends and school needs to a greater degree to acknowledge the assets of the person with deafness and to encourage students who are deaf to have high educational aspirations. By the same token, students with deafness may need professional support, for the social environment often places enormous expectations and demands on those of them who attempt to bridge barriers and initiate new images (e.g., the first person with deafness in a professional area). Such people are often referred to as the "deaf elite", a minority group who have higher education and higher positions in various organizations than the majority of their peers. Belonging to the elite among persons with deafness may result in "personal costs" in terms of less group cohesiveness, and an increased psycho-social isolation within the community of people who are deaf. As the elite are becoming a larger group, individual people who are deaf may feel less isolated in the future.

5. Many students who are deaf do not live in their own family environment during the school years. This is due to the

child's enrolment in a special school for those who are deaf away from the home, and many parents' and siblings' inability to move geographically with the child. Thus the school must take on a greater role compared with regular schools. Personnel require a high level of sign language, and need to foster relations between students in terms of social as well as emotional networks. What makes life difficult for many people with deafness is the lack of knowledge concerning their country's language, and the lack of knowledge concerning the society in which the community members with hearing live. The scholastic requirements in high school must also be increased so that students who are deaf can receive a more realistic appreciation of reality in terms of education, labour-market, economy, social life, relationships and family formation. Students with deafness need social training, including classroom discussions about feelings and relationships, and information about the utilization of sign language interpreters. Furthermore, students who are deaf need secure and stable adult contacts as adequate models of adulthood.

6. In adult years, people with deafness must, on the one hand, be given a fair chance to enter the labour-market, (i.e., information by sign language interpreters about work, the workplace and the work requirements). Employers and employees need, on the other hand, accurate information about deafness and sign language interpretation. Prejudices and negative attitudes from people with hearing still remain in our society and have to be modified. How information about deafness is presented and by whom is vital. Those with hearing need to increase their knowledge about deafness in terms of the problems and difficulties facing persons with deafness and the resources that are available. A research study (Backenroth and Hanson, 1987) showed that clients who were deaf and had strikingly few apparent resources paradoxically had demonstrably rich resources. It is the counsellor's role to cultivate these resources and communicate them within the network. People with deafness also need to increase their knowledge about people who can hear so that they are conscious about similarities and differences. This is important in order for both people

with deafness and with hearing to move closer to each other. The opportunities for interplay and communication depend on reciprocity, on the willingness of both parties to collaborate, and the mutual interest and compliance of both sides in developing understanding, acceptance and cooperation.

7. Employers and employees must realize the necessity for sign language interpretation. There is a striking shortage of interpreters in Sweden today and the demand far exceeds the supply. The interpreter service must be increased in order for people who are deaf to have equal opportunities and participation in society. Recruitment models for potential interpreters must be developed. People with deafness must have access to interpreters in various situations and they must feel secure that interpreters are available. Interpreters, on the other hand, must be well educated in Swedish, sign language, interpreting skills, as well as general knowledge. The education of interpreters needs to be improved while continuing education of initial training should be provided.

8. People who are deaf also need opportunities for further educational and professional retraining. Furthermore, they need opportunities to develop their social network at work with other people with deafness. Thus several people who are deaf need to be employed at the same workplace.

9. Associations for persons with deafness need to initiate more discussion about deafness and impairment in society, as well as raise the consciousness of those who are deaf about attitudes, values, and identity concepts. Further, they can encourage knowledge about relationships, group processes and how people exert influence over one another. In particular they need to sensitize people with deafness to how the "gossip network" in their own community is experienced by individual people with deafness, and what can be done to foster an increased openness, tolerance and cohesiveness. The character of the associations for people with deafness has gradually changed over the years and today represents a far more heterogenous network for members who are deaf. Thus the associations need to reappraise their role for

various groups of members with deafness, enhancing potential changes and implementing new activity groups as a result of these developmental trends. The professional network often neglects the strength of the informal social network. Cooperation between informal and formal networks and the professional network can be fruitful in strengthening the social network of persons with deafness and in enhancing activity and competence in the community of the future. It should be recognized that social networks do not only constitute advantages, but can involve disadvantages in terms of personal costs, including control, overprotection, and less personalized developmental possibilities. Future research needs to investigate the nature of these social networks and identify favourable aspects. People need to know the "how" and "when" of networking as well as the mechanisms which encourage the mobilization of informal support systems which can empower people with deafness through self-help.

REFERENCES

Ahlgren, I. (1978) *Early Linguistic Cognitive Development in the Deaf and Severely Hard of Hearing*. Department of Linguistics, Stockholm University, Stockholm.

Axelsson, M. and Crafoord, E. (1975) *Personlighetsutveckling vid Dovhet. 2: Intervjuer med "Nyckelpersoner" inom Dovomradet*, Psykologexamensarbete, Department of Psychology, Stockholm University, Stockholm.

Auerbach, A.B. (1959) 'What Can Parents Gain from Group Experience?' in *Child Study Association of America, Helping Parents of Handicapped Children - Group Approaches*. Child Study Association of America, New York.

Auerbach, A.B. (1961) 'Group Education for Parents of the Handicapped', *Children, 8*, 135-140.

Award, G. (1978) 'Mental Health Service for the Deaf', *Hospital and Community Psychology, 29*, 674-677.

Backenroth, G. (1975) 'Forskning om Foraldrar', *SDR-Kontakt, 23*, 6-7, 11.

Backenroth, G. (1976) *Att Vara Foraldrar till ett Dovt Barn, Pilotstudie till Projektet; Kristerapeutisk Verksamhet for*

Horande Foraldrar till Dova och Gravt Horselskadade Barn., Psykologexamensarbete, Department of Psychology, Stockholm University, Stockholm.

Backenroth, G. (1978) *Kristerapeutisk Verksamhet for Horande Foraldrar till Dova och Gravt Horselskadade Barn. Delrapport 1: Gruppsamtal med Foraldrar i Stockholm*, Department of Psychology, Stockholm University, Stockholm.

Backenroth, G. (1980) 'Foraldrastodjande Insatser med Terapeutisk Inriktning', Lagesbeskrivning, Stiftelsen for Foraldrasamverkan, DHB-HfR-SDR, Stockholm, (unpublished manuscript).

Backenroth, G. (1983) 'Group Counseling for Parents of Deaf and Hearing Impaired Children', Doctoral Dissertation, Department of Psychology, Stockholm University, Stockholm.

Backenroth, G. (1984a) *Foraldrar till Dova Barn och Deras Livssituation i ett Ferarigt Perspektiv*, 43, Department of Psychology, Stockholm University, Stockholm.

Backenroth, G. (1984b) *Gruppsamtal for Foraldrar till Dova Barn - en Kvantitativ Uppfoljningsstudie*, 44, Department of Psychology, Stockholm University, Stockholm.

Backenroth, G. (1984c) *Foraldrars Accepterande av Horselhandikappet i ett Flerarigt Perspektiv*, 45, Department of Psychology, Stockholm University, Stockholm.

Backenroth, G. (1984d) 'Counselling in Families with a Deaf or Hearing Impaired Child', *International Journal for the Advancement of Counselling, 7,* 267-274.

Backenroth, G. (1986a) *Bilden som Hjalpmedel i Samtal med Foraldrar till Dova och gravt Horselskadade Barn*, 49, Department of Psychology, Stockholm University, Stockholm.

Backenroth, G. (1986b) 'Counselling with the Psycho-socially Isolated Deaf', *International Journal for the Advancement of Counselling, 9,* 125-131.

Backenroth, G. and Hanson, G. (1986) *En Modell for Psykosocialt Rehabiliteringsarbete Bland Barndomsdova*, 48, Department of Psychology, Stockholm University, Stockholm.

Backenroth, G. (1987a) 'The Role of the Family and Society in Providing Favourable Conditions for the Deaf Family Member', Plenary speech presented at IRTAC's (International Round Table for the Advancement of Counselling) Conference in Vienna, July 7, (unpublished manuscript).

Backenroth, G. (1987b) 'Group Support for Parents of Deaf and Hearing Impaired Children', *International Journal Rehabilitation Research, 10,* 324-327.

Backenroth, G. and Borgen, B. (eds) (1987) 'Counselling Disabled

People and their Families', Third International Consultation Report, Rehabilitation International, Vienna, Austria.

Backenroth, G. and Hanson, G. (1987) *Sociala Natverk Bland Dova som Soker Psykologiskt Stod, 50,* Department of Psychology, Stockholm University, Stockholm.

Backenroth, G. (1988) *Personalhandledning for Tolkar som Arbetar Bland Dova, 55,* Department of Psychology, StockholmUniversity, Stockholm.

Backenroth, G. (1989) 'Necessary Prerequisites for Deaf's Self-actualization in a Hearing Society', XXIV International Congress of Psychology in Sydney, *Social Applications and Issues in Psychology, 8,* 251-260.

Baratz, S. and Baratz, J. (1970) 'Early Childhood Intervention: The Social Sciences Base of Institutional Racism', *Harvard Educational Review, 40,* 290-295.

Basilier, T. (1964) 'Surdophrenia. The Psychic Consequences of Acquired Deafness', *Acta Psychiatrica Scandinavica,* supplement, 180, 40, 363-372.

Basilier, T. (1973) *Horseltap og Egentlig Dovhet i Socialpsykiatrisk Perspektiv,* Universitetforlaget, Oslo, Norway.

Bergman, B. (1982) *Studies in Swedish Sign Language,* Department of Linguistics, Stockholm University, Stockholm.

Caplan, R.D. (1981) 'How Social Support Prevents Social Problems in Life Transitions', Presented at the American Psychology Association Conference, Los Angeles, CA (unpublished manuscript).

Cassel, J. (1974) 'Psychosocial Processes and "Stress". Theoretical Formulations', *International Journal of Health Service, 4,* 471-482.

Cassel, J. (1976) 'The Contribution of the Social Environment to Host Resistance', *American Journal of Epidemiology, 104,* 107-123.

Crafoord, E. and Axelsson, M. (1975) *Personlighetsutveckling vid Dovhet. Hur det kanns att vara dov. Riksomfattande Enkat.* Department of Psychology, Stockholm University, Stockholm.

Crafoord, C. (1987) *Den Mojliga och Omojliga Psykiatrin. Utveckling och Erfarenheter av Sektoriserad Psykiatri.* Natur and Kultur, Stockholm.

Denmark, J.C. (1966) 'Mental Illness and Early Profound Deafness', *British Journal of Medical Psychiatry, 39,* 117-124.

Denmark, J.C. and Eldridge, R.W. (1969) 'Psychiatric Services for the Deaf', *The Lancet, Aug. 2,* 259-262.

Drapela, V.J. (1983) *The Counselor as Consultant and Supervisor*, Charles C. Thomas, Springfield, Illinois.

Estroff, S.E. (1983) 'How Social is Psychosocial Rehabilitation?' *Psychosocial Rehabilitation Journal*, 7, 6-20.

Feldman, W. (1981) *Foraldrautbildning i Samtalsgrupp. Handledning for Gruppledare och Foraldrar*, Almqvist and Wiksell, Stockholm.

Fenderson, D.A. (1984) 'Opportunities for Psychologists in Disability Research', *American Psychologist*, 39, 524-528.

Fernlund, K. and Gustafsson, I. (1981) Foraldra-grupper. Upplaggning, Genomforande och Resultat, *Socialstyrelsen: Foraldrar och Barn, nr. 2*.

Fitzgerald, L.F. and Osipow, S.H, (1986) 'An Occupational Analysis of Counseling Psychology. How Special is the Speciality?' *The American Psychologist*, 41, 535-544.

Furth, H.G. (1977) *Tankande Utan Sprak. Dovhet och Inlarning. Ett Psykologiskt Perspektiv*, Wahlstrom and Widstrand, Stockholm.

Garstecki, D.C. (1982) 'Rehabilitation of Hearing-handicapped Elderly Adults', *Ear & Hearing*, 3, 167-172.

Goldman, L. (1976) 'A Revolution in Counseling Research', *Journal of Counseling Psychology*, 23, 543-552.

Goldstein, H. (1986) 'A Cognitive-Humanistic Approach to the Hard-to-reach Client, *Journal of Contemporary Social Work*, 67, 27-36.

Gottlieb, B.H. (1985) 'Social Networks and Social Support: An Overview of Research, Practice, and Policy Implications', *Health Education Quarterly*, 12, 5—22.

Greenblatt, M., Becerra, R. and Serafetinides, E.A. (1982) 'Social Networks and Mental Health: An Overview', *American Journal of Psychiatry*, 139(8), 977-984.

Hoyt, M.F., Siegelman, E.Y. and Schlesinger, H.S. (1981) 'Special Issues Regarding Psychotherapy with the Deaf', *American Journal of Psychiatry*, 138(6), 807-811.

Jongkees, L.B.W. (1983) 'Psychological Problems of the Deaf', *The Annals of Otology, Rhinology and Laryngology*, 92, 8-13.

Levine, E.S. (1976) 'Psychological Contributions', *Volta Review, 78*, 23—33.

Magnusson, D., Duner, A. and Zetterblom, G. (1975) *Adjustment. A Longitudinal Study*. Almqvist and Wiksell, Stockholm.

Magnusson, D. and Endler, N.S. (1976) *Interactional Psychology:*

Present Status and Future Prospects. Department of Psychology, Stockholm University, Stockholm.

Mahapatra, S.B. (1974) 'Deafness and Mental Health: Psychiatric and Psychosomatic Illness in the Deaf', *Acta Psychiatrica Scandinavica 50*, 596-611.

McDowell, J. and Gabel, H. (1981) 'Social Support Among Mothers of Mentally Retarded Children', George Peabody College, Vanderbilt University, (unpublished manuscript).

Meadow, K.P. (1969) 'Self-image, Family Climate and Deafness', *Social Forces, 37*, 428-438.

Menolascino, F.J. and Coleman, R. (1980) 'The Pilot Parent Programme: Helping Handicapped Children Through their Parents', *Child Psychology and Human Development, 1,* 41-48.

Mindel, E.D. and Vernon, McCay (1971) *They Grow in Silence. The Deaf and his Family,* National Association of the Deaf (NAD), Silver Spring, Maryland.

Morrill, W.H., Oetting, E.R. and Hurst, J.C. (1974) 'Dimensions of Counselor Functioning', *Personnel and Guidance Journal, 52,* 354-359.

Norden, K. (1975) 'Psychological Studies of Deaf Adolescents', Doctoral dissertation, Studia Psychologica et Paedagogica Series Altera XXIX. CWK Gleerup, Lund, Sweden.

Norden, K. (1981) 'Learning Processes and Personality Development in Deaf Children', *The American Annals of the Deaf, 126,* 404-410.

Östergren, P.O. (1984) *Socialt Stod och Halsa. En Selekterad Oversikt av Litteraturen inom Omradet 1976-83,* Department of Clinical and Social Medicine, Lund University, Lund Sweden.

Patterson, C.J. (1974) *Relationship Counseling and Psychotherapy,* Harper and Row, New York.

Preisler, G. (1983) 'Deaf Children in Communication. A Study of Communicative Strategies used by Deaf Children in Social Interaction', Doctoral dissertation, Department of Psychology, Stockholm University, Stockholm.

Pyke, J.M. and Littman, S.K. (1982) 'A Psychiatric Clinic for the Deaf', *Canadian Journal of Psychiatry 27,* 384-389.

Raubolt, R.R. (1985) 'Humanistic Analysis: Integrating Action and Insight in Psychotherapy', *Journal of Contemporary Psychotherapy, 15,* 46-56.

Remvig, J. (1969) 'Three Clinical Studies of Deaf-mutism and Psychotherapy, Doctoral dissertation, *Acta Psychiatria, Scandinavia, Supplement, 210,* Munksgaard, Copenhagen, Denmark.

Robertson, S.E. (1988) 'Social Support: Implications for Counselling',

International Journal for the Advancemment of Counselling, 11, 313-321.

Robinson, L.D. (1971) 'Treatment and Rehabilitation of the Mentally Ill Deaf', *Journal of Rehabilitation of the Deaf, 4(3),* 44—52.

Rogers, C.R. (1942) *Counselling and Psychotherapy,* Houghton-Mifflin, Boston.

Rotter, P. (1974) 'Working with Parents of Young Deaf Children', in R.E. Hardy and J.C. Cull (eds), *Educational and Psychological Aspects of Deafness,* Charles C. Thomas, Springfield, Illinois.

Sarason, J.C., Sarason, B.R. and Shearin, E.N. (1986) 'Social Support as an Individual Difference Variable: Its Stability, Origins, and Relational Aspects', *Journal of Personal and Social Psychology, 50,* 845-855.

Schein, J.D. (1983) 'Cognitive and Emotive Aspects of the Deaf Youth's Self-concepts', Paper presented at the 7th World Congress for the Deaf in Palermo, Italy (unpublished manuscript).

Schlesinger, H.S. and Meadow, K.P. (1972) *'Sound and Sign',* University of California Press, Berkeley.

Sigmon, S.B. (1984) 'Interactionist Psychology. A Fourth Force?', *Psychological Reports, 54,* 156.

Solomon, K. (1976) 'The Hard-of-hearing Psychotherapist', *American Journal of Psychotherapy, 30,* 601-607.

Steele, R.L. (1976) 'Humanistic Psychology and Rehabilitation Programs in Mental Hospitals', *American Journal of Occupational Therapy, 6,* 358-361.

Sue, D.W. (1981) *'Counseling the Culturally Different. Theory and Practice',* John Wiley, New York.

Sue, D.W. and Sue, D. (1977) 'Barriers to Effective Cross-cultural Counseling', *Journal of Counseling Psychology, 24,* 420-429.

Sue, D. and Zane, N. (1987) 'The Role of Culture and Cultural Techniques in Psychotherapy. A Critique and Reformulation', *The American Psychologist, 42,* 37-45.

Sussman, A.E. (1983) 'Attitudes Towards Deafness: Psychology's Role, Past, Present and Potential', Paper presented at the 7th World Congress for the Deaf , in Palermo, Italy (unpublished manuscript).

Svedhem, L., Bergerhed, E., Brendler, M., Forsberg, G., Hultkrantz-Jeppson, A., Klefbeck, J., Linner, A., Marklund, K., Martensson, L. and Swaling, J. (1985), *Natverksterapi. Teori och Praktik,* Carlssons, Bokforlag AB, Stockholm.

Thoreson, R.W., and Tully, N.L. (1971) 'Role and Function of the Counselor', in A.E. Sussman and L.G. Stewart (eds), *Counseling with the Deaf People,* New York University School of Education, Deafness Research and Training Centre, New York.

Trotzer, J.P. (1977) *The Counselor and the Group: Integrating Theory, Training, and Practice,* Brooks/Cole, Monterey, California.

Vernon, McCay (1970) 'Potential, Achievement, and Rehabilitation in the Deaf Population', *Rehabilitation Literature, 31*(9), 258-267.

Vernon, McCay (1971) 'Current Status of Counseling with Deaf People', in A.E. Sussman and L.G. Stewart (eds) *Counseling with the Deaf People,* New York University, School Education, Deafness Research and Training Centre, New York.

Vernon, McCay (1972) 'Psychodynamics Surrounding the Diagnosis of the Child's Deafness', *Rehabilitation Psychology., 3,* 127-134.

Vernon, McCay (1975) 'Major Current Trends in Rehabilitation and Education of the Deaf and Hard of Hearing', *Rehabilitation Literature, 36,* 102-107.

Williams, B.R. and Sussman, A.E. (1971) 'Social and Psychological Problems of Deaf People', in A.E. Sussman and L.G. Stewart (eds) *Counseling with the Deaf People.* New York University School of Education, Deafness Research and Training Centre, New York.

Chapter Eleven

SOME CHALLENGES TO COUNSELLING
IN THE FIELD OF DISABILITIES

Roy I. Brown

INTRODUCTION

One important issue in rehabilitation raised during the last two decades is that of quality of life. It is increasingly quoted as a new vision of rehabilitation enabling us to abandon some of our previous concepts and look at rehabilitation and its allied functions in a new and perhaps expanded fashion. It is perhaps best seen as one of a number of developmental blocks – a move from previously held views and values to a slightly different conceptualization. As such, many of the ideas associated with quality of life have been employed in the field for some while, yet it can be argued that a quality of life model enables rehabilitation counsellors to view their tasks in a broader format and to look more closely at the perceptions of their clients in the process of rehabilitation.

Although some have argued that there are differing views about a definition of quality of life, it would seem that there are some commonly held views concerning the components which make up quality of life. These components suggest a broad definition (Brown, Bayer and MacFarlane, 1989; Goode, 1988; Parmenter, 1987, 1988) involving all aspects of a person's life. Perhaps more important, quality of life is directed towards areas in which consumers indicate that they wish to improve their function. However, quality health care is frequently seen as a judgement made by health care professionals, and for the clinician, diagnosis leads to opinions on the nature of physical rehabilitation. A study of individuals who have been rehabilitated often leads to suggestions that the clients' views of the rehabilitation process are different from those of the professionals who provide the service.

It is apparent from Halpern, Close and Nelson (1986) and Parmenter (1988) that quality of life is made up of a wide range of components. There is some agreement amongst these authors on the components of quality of life including the major dimensions such as leisure, social, home living, vocational and educational skills studied by Brown and others. Results reflect directly or indirectly that emotional perceptions and concerns need to constitute an important part of any quality of life model.

Both clients and their sponsors (often spouses or parents) need to be asked questions about life for the individual concerned. Questions involving areas of improvement or deterioration are critical – for example, perceived deterioration in behaviour or specific skills while attending a rehabilitation centre may have profound effects on motivation and self-image. Questions relating to perceived quality of environment or one's own perception of health are important. An appraisal by the consumer of worries and anxieties, perceived needs for emotional support or for desired changes in professional or personal relationships should also be included (for further examples see Brown and Bayer, 1991). Such information can provide knowledge about functioning, environmental structure and professional skills along with direction for change and improvement.

The models referred to above are holistic, that is they involve all areas of an individual's functioning or interests. Most models recognize that objective measures involve only one, and possibly at times, a small component of individual functioning – subjective and personal processes represent a growing area of interest. There are many issues relating to mind-body interaction and consciousness that have not yet been sufficiently explored nor subjected to measurement. It seems quite possible that in certain types of disability consciousness or limitations to consciousness may be important in terms of rehabilitation. Conscious awareness of all aspects of disability are important from the consumer's perspective if the individual is going to gain control over aspects of functioning. The counsellor cannot help to bring this about unless she or he also is aware of these same processes. For these reasons measurement of the more subjective and personal aspects of quality of life becomes critical.

Brown *et al.*, (1989) have defined quality of life as follows:

> The discrepancy between a person's achieved and
> unmet needs and desires. This refers to the
> subjective, or perceived, and objective assessment
> of an individual's domains (p. 57). The extent to
> which an individual increasingly controls aspects of
> life regardless of original baseline (p. 58).

Although this definition does not imply replacing
objective assessment, it does involve increased attention to
subjective aspects or perceptions of and by the client, which may
be critical to the rehabilitation process. This is essential in the
authors' quality of life model. This is not to say that counsellors
and others have not sought the opinion of persons with
disabilities in the past, but perhaps suggests that such a model
has not played a rigorous or central part in the process of
rehabilitation. Brown, Bayer and Brown (1988, 1992) have
indicated in their quality of life questionnaire, that the subjective
areas involve broad aspects of life and are not limited to the
areas thought to surround and encompass disability. It should
be recognized that what appears to be the disability in the eye of
the professional may be something quite different from the
point of view of the client. Brown *et al.*, (1989) have pointed out
that professionals may believe that clients need to attain or
retain specific standards of rehabilitation in their lifestyle
relating to, for example, perceived safety, communication, or
mobility. An examination of quality of life including subjective
perceptions of behaviours and lifestyle may indicate that
although attaining professionally based rehabilitative criteria,
the individual still feels unrehabilitated. A person may, for
example, feel unsafe or unwell despite the clinical perception of
the client held by the professional. It is suggested that this
personal subjectivity may constitute a reality which is way
beyond that of the objective measures or formal results obtained
through traditional assessments. Sometimes the client's
perceptions of performance may be higher than objective
assessment warrants. Here again such discrepant information is
relevant and opens up opportunities for counselling. Again the
concern is not whether the client's response is objectively right
or wrong. The counsellor uses the information as part of the

process to bring about change. Indeed, recent evidence (Brown, Bayer and Brown, 1992) suggests that during the process of rehabilitation counselling, clients' and sponsors' views tend to come much closer, increasing the chances of success and ease of subsequent intervention. This is relevant to a full understanding of the rehabilitation process.

MEASUREMENT OF QUALITY OF LIFE

It is has normally been assumed that objective measures in assessment are more easily undertaken than subjective ones. Objective measures are capable of replication and are subject to evaluation of reliability and validity. They can be evaluated against other variables which may be seen as important indicators of change. Yet such evaluations, despite their objective reliability, have not necessarily produced results which satisfy clients, and the measures cannot be seen as a comprehensive evaluation of consumer performance or perception. It is these concerns which make it necessary to go one stage further and define the areas of quality of life from the individual's point of view, and to recognize that subjective behaviours and perceptions may have a validity which is intrinsic and fundamental to the functioning of the individual.

For example, many consumers in rehabilitation centres note that personal and emotional needs are rarely met. Many clients may not have the verbal abilities to define or confine their emotional problems, and it behooves the counsellor to recognize that both verbal and non-verbal techniques may be necessary to assess these aspects of concern. In more severe cases of disability it should be recognized that visual and tactile assessment of quality of life through observation may represent the major and most important methods of clarifying needs and choices. Such information is critical for selecting and building ecologically sound rehabilitation environments.

Sponsors, that is parents or partners, need also to be involved in evaluation of quality of life. They too may be involved in assessment of quality of life in instances where the individual cannot express needs. However, it must be recognized that sponsors may also make assumptions about individuals' lives which are incorrect and do not necessarily address the needs of the individual. For such reasons it is apparent that there must be much more careful research and examination of the subjective and perceptual aspects of quality of life from the perspective of the individual consumer. The discussion above raises issues relating to self-image, empowerment and choice.

CHOICE AND QUALITY OF LIFE

Quality of life models involve client choice and accept, as Brown *et al.*, (1991) and Goode (1988) have indicated, the notion that the client's wishes must be paramount in the design of any rehabilitation process. The above authors suggest that the client's choice must be accepted regardless of its apparent relevance or irrelevance to the client's functioning. However, Brown *et al.* (1991) also argue that the role of the professional rehabilitation counsellor, once the notion of choice is accepted, is to structure skilfully the environment and ensure that counselling enables individuals to function effectively in the domain of their choice. This may mean moving gradually, in a step-wise fashion, to the fulfilment of such choices or goals. It may result in changes in choice by the client. The important issue is acceptance of the individual's perceptions and choices. Such acceptance is critical to self-image and motivation.

Professionals have argued that choice, in many cases of disability, may not be a realistic or a reliable function. Individuals may change their choices over fairly short periods of time. This, for example, is particularly noted in the field of mental handicap, but is also apparent where aging is linked to disability, and in the field of mental health. But this ignores the role or frequency of change in choice in the populations without disabilities. It is argued that too many professional procedures overlook the input that the client can have in terms of controlling the rehabilitation process. Very often, where client choice has been noted, as in individual planning procedures, it has been associated with involving the individual in group meetings with a number of professional personnel. This represents an unsatisfactory use of personnel. It is also counter-indicated by a quality of life model, since most individuals cannot cope, or at least limit their verbal responses (Brown and

Hughson, 1987) in such situations, and are inhibited or are inappropriate in terms of processing their ideas and wishes. This leads to the need for a central planner, manager or organizer who is responsible for developing the procedures of rehabilitation in a manner which is consistent with the goals put forward by the client and the overt preference demonstrated by the client. It also provides a meaningful role for a broker (Collier, 1989).

Few studies on choice have been carried out with children or elderly persons with disabilities and it is also recognized that many workers in the field believe that consumers or clients are not capable of making choices, which are safe and in the individual's clinical or treatment interests. It may be important in this context to give some examples.

> A woman in her forties wishes to leave hospital. She has had a stroke and is now non-ambulatory, spending her days in a wheelchair. She has difficulties feeding, but nevertheless wishes to live on her own. The hospital staff indicate that left on her own she is likely to have an accident, get into difficulties and probably die.

Such perceptions and statements often inhibit individuals from making or following through with their choices. The same views may be supported by relatives and friends, who are also concerned about safety and longevity. However, the individual needs to make a choice. While realistic concerns need to be discussed, professional personnel, particularly the core counsellor, should provide the means whereby the barriers to fulfilling choice are dealt with in a direct manner and are removed through joint problem solving strategies. In the example given, advocates or support workers could be involved in solving the problem of where the individual can live independently, under circumstances where she or he can make rapid contact (e.g., by the use of an electronic device) in an emergency. Prosthetic devices can be so arranged that a person can have independence and privacy.

Such an approach also provides the counsellor with a further role. Most rehabilitation services are predicated on administrative procedures which are largely hierarchical. They assume a reporting process and a bureaucracy which makes assumptions about "the best interests of the client" when the system really applies general rules which often result in client care, least bother for personnel and meet certain administrative, economic, and political ends which are said to be in the interests of cost efficiency. If these rules and procedures could be modified through the development of non-hierarchical systems of management, many individuals with disabilities could probably grow to function more effectively. This occurred in the example given, with the support of advocates but with great resistance from the professional personnel. The woman now leads a life of her choice under what most would regard as challenging circumstances, but where needs of personal privacy, control and choice are met.

INDIVIDUALIZED FUNDING AND QUALITY OF LIFE

Recent concepts outlined in a variety of reports (e.g., Brassard Committee, 1989) suggest that society is beginning to have some understanding of the need to individualize funding. This means attaching funds to an individual or his or her representatives and allowing the individual to contract for specific services, thus encouraging the development of more versatile and personal/highly professional forms of service. The counsellor has both professional and policy making roles in such situations. He or she must develop or coordinate procedures for specific clients who require rehabilitation, but must also advocate through the system, for changes in management structure and policy and the implementation of client and rehabilitative choice. The counsellor may need to work with a broker who is knowledgeable about the array of services. This approach is perhaps a slightly different one from that claimed for many practices. The counsellor's attempts to gain insight into the client's perceptions and provide accepted intervention by means of professional procedures. At the same time the counsellor helps the individual to see him or herself in a new light, but far more importantly, the counsellor is there to learn and understand how and why an individual makes particular quality of life choices. The counsellor's knowledge and skill aim to bring about client fulfilment through careful negotiation within the service system, through contracting between service and client and advocacy on behalf of the client.

The arguments above are based on a quality of life model, and use the types of objective and subjective data that are now feasible. These include clinical knowledge relating to the functioning of individuals with different forms of handicap. Some examples follow.

A man was amputated below the knees as a result of a railway accident. Hospitalization following successful amputation included counselling which involved the recommendation that he should consider making plans for a new job in a new setting. He had previously been a manual worker and this was now no longer a feasible proposition. Following the accident, marriage breakdown occurred and his wife moved away taking their daughter with her. This separation was, from the client's perspective, the critical aspect of the accident, not losing his limbs. Increasing pressure was put on him to seek work by bringing the issue to his attention regularly, and with an indication that he would make speedy adaptation if he took this important step. In a tape recording he indicated that he felt unable to do this until he had resolved "in his own mind" the emotional void that was now created by the absence of wife and daughter. There was no evidence that this issue had been perceived by the rehabilitation staff as a major, let alone central issue to rehabilitation. They recognized the concrete and physical aspects of disability, but were unaware of the predominant concern of the individual involving what he perceived as the central emotional and personal issues in his life. It may have been correct that the change in work style would have resolved some of his problems. But it would probably have been much more effective to recognize the personal issues which were seen by the individual as central. In doing so the components and timing of different aspects of rehabilitation would have been changed.

This example raises some important points about rehabilitation and illustrates some of the perceptual changes created by a quality of life model. The issues of choice and subjective perception contained in the example are readily apparent. Further, the idea that the rehabilitation should not necessarily focus primarily or immediately on the concrete and obvious issue which is readily perceived by rehabilitation personnel can also be recognized.

Perhaps even more fundamental is the presenting problems or disabilities perceived as rehabilitation issues. The problems which occur after physical accidents may in part be exacerbated and may be dominated by issues which were taking place prior to what we conveniently call the accident or precipitating cause of disability. It is important to recognize that effective health and optimum functioning may only be recognized when we drop the idea of specific rehabilitation in order to deal much more comprehensively with the holistic challenges facing the individual.

In such a personalized model, there is need for a case manager who is a worker skilled in counselling, but with sufficient practical expertise to develop and to coordinate procedures at the front-line level. Such an individual will operate in the person's natural environments – home, leisure, work and community. Brown *et al.*, (1988, 1991) have pointed out the virtues of moving "rehabilitation" into the home environment and local community. Such movement has, in most cases, the advantage of retaining familiar structures for dealing with realistic problems in realistic settings. Further, much of rehabilitation can only work when persons who live with the individual see the nature of change and relearning and undergo adaptations themselves. They can then become more motivated and thus cope with problems or issues that arise, for they now feel part of the recovery system.

In another example, a father who suffered a stroke returned home from hospital. He had lost speech and considerable motor function at the time of the accident. Prior to hospitalization the individual had wished to build a patio deck. When he left the hospital for home his surgeon and his wife considered this wish inappropriate. There were concerns over care, inability to communicate, apparent loss of motivation, and disorganized behaviours. However, despite little language a rehabilitation practitioner working directly in the home, who accepted the proposition that the individual still wished to build his patio, was able, by providing simple aids plus some manual support, to enable the individual to carry out his task successfully. Not only was this a source of some amazement to the surgeon, but it also surprised the client's wife, who now recognized that her husband was no longer incompetent, despite severe restriction in a number of functions such as language and motor control. She could see that with certain types of support her spouse could function effectively. The process described resulted in an increase in the consumer's motivation, positive growth in self-image and improvement in language and motor skills. Obviously in such clinical reports there can be argument about the causes of change, yet studies indicate that perception of self, along with active success can affect motivation and become key factors in the rehabilitation process.

Brown *et al.*, (1989) have shown that the perceptions of most individuals with mental handicap are accurate including their personal views about personal inadequacy, and progress or deterioration. When they are given choice and control of the learning situation – both the activity and environment – they frequently make dramatic changes in behaviour, in some cases to such an extent, that the individual is no longer recognized as having a disability (Brown *et al.*, 1991). This view is supported by those of Parmenter (1988) and De Jong (1981) who believe society's view of disability acts to encapsulate the individual in a static and uncompromising environment which holds that individual in a state of handicap. Goode (1988) also presents similar arguments. By taking over controls from society and its agents, and placing them in the hands of the consumer, major and positive changes in development can occur.

But there are other major effects. For example, through a quality of life model, our language in describing disability may also be changed. Is an individual with some memory problems, as a result of a bullet wound, necessarily any more a case of disability than someone in their late fifties who is now becoming forgetful. The conclusions we draw results from relative judgments and expectations. It seems likely that people in their late fifties largely recognize their increasing difficulty with retaining new information, but we do not suggest that such a person has a disability even though he or she may show some discrepancy with previous functioning levels. The concern, then, is what is the nature of disability and what is the nature of compensatory assets. For the male in his fifties an asset may be experience and mature judgment. For the woman with a head injury it may be control to exercise choice in her environment. How should we view people who attend counselling within clinics, hospitals or schools? Should we dismiss the notion of disability and replace it with a concept of variability in performance with recognized deficits and assets? Our role as counsellors is to enable the individual to function as effectively as possible in the domains which he or she personally sees as critical to a competent life style.

The above view, if taken seriously, results in a questioning of some of the strongly held notions about the purposes of rehabilitation. For example, bodies, such as Workers Compensation, consider that returning to work and/or replacement work is critical to the rehabilitation process. To this end, funds and welfare are directed. But many individuals have indicated that return to work is not their major wish, nor their major concern, within the rehabilitation process either after an accident or after suffering long-term disability. Although such issues become less of a conceptual concern once individuals have reached retirement age, the notion of accepting an individual's own value system and self-conceptualization has largely been ignored.

Despite our concerns over the employment needs of people with disabilities, Day (1989), Brown *et al.*, (1989) and others have underlined the importance of leisure time within the so-called rehabilitation process. Their evidence suggests that individuals who are vocationally successful have developed their leisure time skills to a greater degree. This raises the potential importance of leisure and recreational activity as a rehabilitation process. Nash (1954) has indicated that four levels of leisure activity exist and although these are somewhat arbitrary, they range over observer, social, physical and self-actualizing types of involvement. It is apparent that the latter two areas, and to some degree the second, are ill-developed or have become under-used in many individuals who have had traumatic or long-standing disabilities. Indeed, fairly recent data from the United States suggests that many people who have disabilities also have a very low level of leisure activities. This relates particularly to physical, social and self-actualizing activities. It does appear that those who have a higher and more broadly based leisure style find their way back to employment much more rapidly.

Data, much from client recordings, often underline the desire to improve leisure of one's choice. There is also evidence that exposure to leisure of a varied nature may improve performance in a wide range of areas, particularly health, physical stamina, motivation and self-image (Emes and Ferris, 1986). Counsellors should be aware of such information and become actively involved in assisting individuals to develop skills and activities in a range of recreation areas based on interests and choice. Although it can be argued that members of the general population vary their leisure interests over their life span across the four areas, there is clear evidence that amongst persons with disabilities that the balance of different types of activities is likely to be more discrepant with an accent on observer activities. The effects of this have already been described. But, in addition, the lack of more advanced leisure activities means limitation of opportunities for social involvement, planning and development.

It is clear in certain types of disability that aspects of abstract conceptualization such as forward planning strategies, become underdeveloped and under-utilized and this is of major concern. The role of catalytic activation of individuals with disabilities is also frequently overlooked. Much time has been spent in the past attempting to enable individuals to function more effectively by learning specific skills. This is often seen as a primary role of rehabilitation centres particularly in relation to work skills. It is argued that behavioural intervention and specific skill strategies, which can improve motor and vocational performance have their place, but it is suggested that individuals will perform more effectively once their motivation system has been activated. Motivation levels can change when there is development of self-interest, empowerment and goal directedness. Much of the work in Brown *et al.*, (1991) appears to reflect this principle. It was through the counsellor working closely with the client in practical situations that the individual became able to develop choice and empowerment. This was initiated by accepting choices by the client, and showing how these could be achieved. These choices were, in the first instance, often of minor significance or, to an outside observer, unimportant. At times, they seemed impractical. In rehabilitation they represent catalytic first steps in rejuvenation. In this context behaviour management involving specific learning strategies has an important but secondary role. The development and activation of choice can only take place when appropriate environments for their development and application are available. Thus, the relearning of skills in a sheltered workshop or hospital is unlikely to develop efficiently, or transfer as effectively as possible because the natural environment in which such skills are deployed is not present. If the individual is in a natural environment (home or work or leisure), the rehabilitation process may still fail, but there is then an opportunity to examine ways in which the environment can be modified or behaviour can be adapted to the circumstances. This readily demonstrates the importance of ecological assessment.

FROM THE CONSUMER — A PERSONAL VIEW OF COUNSELLING

At this stage an argument has been put forward for reconceptualizing the nature of rehabilitation in the behavioural, social and educational contexts. Choice, involving client perception, where the rehabilitation practitioner becomes a processor of rehabilitation choice, is critical. Strategies based on choice have direct relevance for rehabilitation agencies and training of personnel. Such a model also provides challenges for policy, management and administration which need to be reoriented to client perception and choice rather than the goals of agency, society (e.g, re-employment) or professionals. But the argument has been largely based on recent research – what do clients see as the role of the rehabilitation counsellor?

The author collected views about the counselling process from a number of people with various disabilities. However, no attempt was made to classify the types of disability or even note the age of the individuals other than to note all were adults. Rather than keep to traditional questions, it was thought more important to provide relevant questions to be answered by people experiencing a wide range of physical, emotional and allied disorders. The major responses can be classified along the following lines, and reflect to some degree the issues raised earlier.

1. *Clients expect the rehabilitation counsellor to be knowledgeable about rehabilitation.*
   The rehabilitation counsellor should be able to answer basic questions relating to most aspects of rehabilitation in a simple and direct fashion, and should be able to call on a wide range of relevant knowledge of specific value to a particular individual. This very much underlines the argument put forward by Brown *et al.*, (1989) that rehabilitation practitioners should be generically trained so that they are aware of a wide range of disabilities. Individuals generally do not manifest one disability and if one accepts the arguments made earlier, despite a particular classification or label, a very different type or interaction of handicaps may be seen as relevant from the client's perspective.

2. *It is expected that the counsellor has a wide and practical experience of disabilities.*
   If counsellors are to be effective, they must have observed disability in a variety of forms and be knowledgeable about the practical implications of these disabilities in natural environments. Some consumers feel that counsellors who do not themselves have a disability, handicap the development of constructive rehabilitation processes. But even when this view is not put forward, consumers do expect the counsellor to have had experience in working in natural and effective ways in the processes of rehabilitation. This suggests that in order to be an effective rehabilitation

counsellor a number of years of experience in the front-line area is absolutely essential, and much of this should be in community and home environments, rather than sheltered workshops, specialist agencies, etc.

3. *The counsellor should be effective over a wide range of life domains.*
   This should include employment and life skills, though not be limited to these. This also stresses the importance of a widely oriented counselling process for adults which is not focused on vocational rehabilitation alone. Such resources are expected within the same counsellor, underscoring the notion of a keyworker.

4. *Counselling requires that practitioners be skilled in recognition of body and facial language.*
   Clients perceive this to be critically important. This applies to formally trained counsellors and also to others such as social workers, rehabilitation practitioners, occupational therapists and so on, who employ counselling as part of their professional expertise.
   People with disabilities watch for body signs and facial language including, for example, signs of boredom in the counsellor. Lack of interest is often assumed from the way the counsellor looks or the way he or she moves. It is apparent from many of the responses, that individuals felt they had experienced a range of behaviours from their counsellors which were unacceptable – yawning, laughing, and moving inappropriately.

5. *The counsellor should have a sense of humour.*
   This was recognized as an important factor and is of particular interest because other studies (Brown *et al.*, 1989) have noted the same interest amongst clients with developmental disabilities. A sense of humour is recognized as a positive personality characteristic amongst counsellors. For example, a sense of humour in a residential counsellor was seen as an important aspect of behaviour by young men and women with developmental disabilities (Brown *et al.*, 1989). This is not always thought of as an important characteristic when selecting a rehabilitation counsellor or rehabilitation counselling student.

6. *The physical relationship of the client to the counsellor during the interview is seen as critical.*
Most clients noted that they wanted counsellors to be at arm's length, but some also did not want a table between the counsellor and themselves. However, it is suspected that these wishes are somewhat idiosyncratic, and clients may prefer different types of environments and also prefer different settings during the counselling process. The client's perception and selection of such situations should be a factor that is recognized with provision made for client choice.

7. *Many individuals spoke of limited time for counselling.*
Consumers noted that counsellors were often unable to provide sufficient time to deal with the issues that were raised. Many clients felt that their needs were much wider and greater than the specific conditions for which they had been referred. Although they often saw counsellors as effective, clients noted frequently that counsellors had inadequate time for follow-up. Thus, some problems and difficulties which arose received no attention, and clients perceived themselves as unable to manage the resulting stress. This is consistent with the Brown and Hughson (1987) argument that individuals regress once they are in new situations or slightly new concerns arise. At such times clients need ready access to their counsellor or practitioner if they are to stabilize and develop. Without such availability, it is likely that rehabilitation efficacy is diminished. Further, a time-limited process may also not be cost effective. If the rehabilitation counselling process is started, sufficient resources must be provided to ensure it is continued and available at times of need. This means further examination of how counselling services are supplied and funded over time. For example, information about recovery from brain injury (Smith, 1983) suggests that in some instances ten to fifteen years may not be too long a time before psychological recovery from brain injury is observable. This has major implications for counselling.

8. *The development and maintenance of positive self-image is*

seen as critical by consumers, and the effect of the counsellor on self-image is perceived as dramatic.

From the arguments made earlier, it is believed that the recovery of positive self-image may be critical to successful rehabilitation, regardless of the apparent physical condition of the individual. Thus some people with massive injury may, because of positive self-image, make effective recovery while those with relatively minor injuries and poor self-image may make poor adjustment. Although this has long been recognized, the nurturing and development of positive self image has been given relatively little attention in rehabilitation as a developed intervention strategy.

9. *The counsellor needs to recognize that the critical aspects of disability perceived by the consumer may be different from the primary disability presented through referral.*
   Many of the issues that the client wishes to discuss with his or her counsellor and perceives as critical are not concerned with the formal aspects of disability, but centre on other issues which may predate or may result from the primary precipitating disability. It is legitimate that these are seen as aspects and possibly primary aspects of the counselling and rehabilitation process by the rehabilitation team. This should be the choice of the consumer.

10. *Good listening skills are seen as a major counselling attribute.*
    It is apparent that many persons with disabilities do not think counsellors practice or develop their listening skills. Individuals who responded to the questionnaire indicated that they felt they were interrupted by counsellors before they had finished ideas while one said "Don't prepare your (counsellor) response until I finish my statement". The general issue is a request for positive feedback after effective listening. Although this represents an aspect of common counselling knowledge which is taught and practised within many counselling programmes, a number of clients did not see this as being practised by the counsellor within their sessions. Counsellors need to monitor continually their practice. It should also be recognized that many professionals providing counselling are untrained in these skills.

11. *Clients saw the need for a variety of counsellors, but underlined the importance of qualifications within counselling.*
Even now, many practitioners who use counselling may not have had formal training in this area. This is true of a wide range of rehabilitation practitioners. Often it may not be a major component in the courses provided to other rehabilitation practitioners, who find themselves in need of counselling skills. Further, individuals who do undertake formal counselling education may not continue to update their skills or ensure that they are continuing to practise their skills over their professional lives.

12. *Individuals felt that it was critical that the counsellor enable the client to increase motivation to take action.*
This was raised by several clients and is seen as a critical issue in the arguments made above. Motivation and its perception are the basis of change. Promoting motivation, therefore, becomes the basis of effective counselling.

13. *Voice skills are often seen as poor, being described as "uninteresting" and "monotonous".*
It is important that professionals receive feedback in training and during their careers concerning voice presentation. Conveying interest, empathy and other behavioural attitudes relate to the way the individual speaks. Many clients may respond to the voice characteristics as much or more than to the context of the verbal statements.

14. *Counsellors are not given adequate time to see their client, or have a large caseload, which reduces the possibility of being involved for long periods at a time with any one client.*
The emotional bond that can develop between counsellor and client can be critical to the rehabilitation process. Many of the issues raised relate to the process of counsellor selection and also the development of counselling skills during training.
    If services and individual counsellors are concerned over outcome, adequate time must be provided. Both quality and equality of the rehabilitation counselling process are critical,

and clients need to have more input and control over both of these aspects of rehabilitation. For example, they should have choice over duration of counselling session and expect to be responded to positively regarding the total duration of the rehabilitation process. This does not mean that the counsellor cannot mediate in this situation, for he or she needs to be controller of the process, but it is intended to indicate that clients should be empowered to take precedence over rigid administration or management procedures.

It might be appropriate to ask consumers to become involved in the selection of counselling students. Such clients might play a role in the development of courses and the evaluation of programmes. These are not practices commonly utilized in university or college departments, yet the clients represent the major stakeholders. A wide range of persons have disabilities and are competent to carry out such procedures. Within some school education systems, lay personnel are provided with an opportunity to interview teachers who may become teachers. There is no reason why this should not be done within the rehabilitation process for the selection of a wide range of counsellors. Yet most rehabilitation services do not employ such approaches. This again represents an important aspect of an applied quality of life model for the clients (or their representatives) who begin to exert their perceptions and their choices. Indeed, it would be prudent to encourage persons with disabilities to receive counselling education and enter employment and teaching. They are considerably under-represented in these areas.

15. *Counsellors must be in a position to help their clients deal with issues that arise in working or living with persons without disabilities.*
   Aspects of ridicule were of major concern to clients. Some maintained this occurred fairly frequently. This underscores the lack of many in society to empathize with individuals' disabilities. Counsellors should practice in situations (i.e., natural environments) where they can witness such ridicule or difficulties between persons with and without disabilities and learn more about how to cope with them.

A number of other issues were cited by consumers.

Individuals needed help in "accepting their past". This tends to support the argument that primary rehabilitation counselling may not necessarily relate to the precipitating or primary cause of disability as initially seen by rehabilitation workers, but to other aspects of experience existing prior to the disability.

Some consumers were concerned that suggestions made by counsellors were unrealistic. This is particularly interesting in the light of the suggestion that counsellors should accept the choices of the individual rather than make goal demands on the consumers. Issues relating to ethical and confidentiality matters were also raised. For example, some noted that counsellors should not contact family members without permission. This is again a choice issue which in most circumstances should be decided by the consumer. Some consumers indicated need for counselling over budgeting resources, appropriate clothing, or how to develop good eye-to-eye contact. Some stated that offering the client something to drink when he or she arrived at a counselling session facilitated a positive environment. All of these are client choice issues. Indeed the issues discussed in this chapter underline the importance of teaching student counsellors about quality of life assessment, and providing education in how to mediate choice and allied quality of life issues, while ensuring the consumer has increased control of life issues both within and surrounding the rehabilitation process.

The list of areas raised beyond the primary disability included problems in human relations, issues relating to divorce, assisting the individual with communication, helping the individual obtain employment, and guidance in developing positive relations with others. Other areas involved social and emotional concerns and need for community support, and help in using community resources. The list of items stresses the number of issues not concerning employment or even the presenting diability. Rehabilitation counsellors need to recognize the diversity of need which involves or surrounds or predates disability. Recreation, separating oneself from a situation, and ability to analyze situations before reacting, were also seen as important aspects of the counselling role, but recognition of the individual's value and his or her role in a particular situation were seen as critical. Individuals were often quite practical in their needs, for example, cooking, cleaning, personal care, budgeting, and living arrangements. Clients needed their counsellor to understand them in a non-judgemental manner. Trust should be engendered, but the counsellor often has to respond to practical needs such as helping to find a place to live, job-hunting or accompanying the individual on a task, plus providing peer support and help in making appointments. These stress the versatility and practicality expected of the counsellor. In one case an individual indicated the person should be of senior age so that he or she "understood from life experience". In another case it was indicated that a comparable age to the client was important. It might be wise to provide a list of the characteristics wanted by the consumer before a formal counsellor is selected. A variety of counsellors might be made available in order that the individual might choose his or her counsellor. Such a system has been recommended and practiced by Fewster and Curtis (1989). One client noted that the counsellor needs to build "on little things" for individuals will not show personal attributes right away. The need for counselling over emotional issues, education, alcoholism in the home, and stress factors were also mentioned. Listening, without interrupting or interpreting, is seen as important by some clients. The need to know whether body language is important to a client seems necessary. One client noted that for visually impaired people, body language could not be read and therefore was inappropriate.

Most consumers work to improve their quality of life, and much of this they see relating to their ability to interact effectively with their environment. This is the purpose of rehabilitation counselling.

CONCLUSION

The above underline some of the issues that might be considered from the point of view of a quality of life model of rehabilitation counselling. It is not intended to be comprehensive, but is an attempt to raise some of the concerns from the client's perspective and their relevance to a preferred model. Many of the procedures are ones already used by counsellors and are certainly ones that should be addressed by students. Despite this, many counsellors, over the course of a professional lifetime, may come to ignore some of these attributes. As time passes, so clients become more sophisticated, and wish to see more sensitive skills within the individual who is their counsellor. The idea that persons with disabilities should be involved in the selection of student counsellors and in the appointment of counsellors to services seems to be important. The involvement of persons with disabilities in the evaluation of counselling programmes within tertiary education, and also in client settings also seems to be appropriate.

The chapter has underlined some of the issues relating to an holistic approach to rehabilitation counselling seen from a quality of life perspective. While recognizing that the client should be the selector of rehabilitation goals, it is stressed that the professional counsellor is the processor of goals, who functions at a very practical and intimate level with the clients in his or her natural environment. It is recognized that there will be enormous variability, not just in relation to disability, but more importantly between clients and within clients over time. These are factors which need to be borne in mind throughout the counselling process by all those who have face-to-face contact with clients, thus stressing the need to be sensitive to clients' personal characteristics and wishes in the development of their rehabilitation programmes.

REFERENCES

Brassard, R. (1989) *Claiming My Future: A Person with a Mental Disability - Today and Tomorrow.* Report of the Brassard Committee to the Government of Alberta.

Brown, R.I. and Bayer, M.B. (1991) *The Personal Rehabilitation Questionnaire - A Guide to an Individual's Quality of Life Through Personal Perception*, (in press).

Brown, R.I., Bayer, M.B. and Brown, P.M. (1988) 'Quality of Life: A Challenge for Rehabilitation Agencies', *Australia and New Zealand Journal of Developmental Disabilities*, 14(3/4), 189–199.

Brown, R.I., Bayer, M.B. and MacFarlane, C. (1989) 'Quality of Life Amongst Handicapped Adults', in R.I. Brown (ed), *Quality of Life for Handicapped People*, Croom Helm, London.

Brown, R.I., Bayer, M.B. and MacFarlane, C., (1989) *Rehabilitation Programmes: Performance and Quality of Life of Adults with Developmental Handicaps*, Lugus, Ontario.

Brown, R.I., Bayer, M.B. and Brown, P.M. (1992) *Empowerment and Developmental Handicaps: Choices and Quality of Life,* Captus, North York, Ontario.

Brown, R.I. and Hughson, E.A. (1987) *Behavioural and Social Rehabilitation and Training,* Wiley, New York.

Close, D.W. (1988) 'Rehabilitation Research and Training Center in Mental Retardation,' in R.I. Brown (ed) *Quality of Life for Handicapped People,* Croom Helm, London.

Collier, M. (1989) *Right to Choose,* videotape, Yale Town Productions, Vancouver.

Day, H. I. (1989) 'Quality of Life of People with Disabilities', *Keynote address, Fourth Canadian Congress of Rehabilitation,* Toronto.

DeJong, G. (1981) *Environmental Accessibility and Independent Living Outcomes. Directions for Disability Policy and Research,* University Center for International Rehabilitation, Michigan State University.

Emes, C. and Ferris, B. (1986) *Physical Activities Amongst Activity-limited and Disabled Canadians,* Ottawa, Fitness Canada.

Fewster, G. and Curtis, J. (1989) 'Creating Options: Designing a Radical Children's Mental Health Programmes', in R.I. Brown and M. Chazan (eds), *Learning Difficulties and Emotional Problems,* Detselig Enterprises Ltd., Calgary, Alberta.

Goode, David A. (1988) *Discussing Quality of Life: The Process and Findings of the Work Group on Quality of Life for Persons with Disabilities.* Mental Retardation Institute, A University Affiliated Programmes, Westchester County Medical Center in Affiliation with New York Medical College, Valhalla, New York.

Halpern, A.S., Close, D.W. and Nelson, D.J. (1986) *On My Own. The Impact of Semi-independent Living Programmess for Adults with Mental Retardation,* Paul H. Brookes, Baltimore, Maryland.

Nash, J.B. (1954) *Philosophy of Recreation and Leisure,* William C. Brown Co., Dubuque, Iowa.

Parmenter, T.R. (1987) *Quality of Life of People with Physical Disabilities,* MacQuarie University. Mimeo.

Parmenter, T.R. (1988) 'An Analysis of the Dimensions of Quality of Life for People with Physical Disabilities', in R.I. Brown (ed), *Quality of Life for Handicapped People,* Croom Helm, London.

Smith, A. (1983) 'Clinical Psychological Practice and Principles of Neuropsychological Assessment', in E.C. Walker (ed) *Handbook of Clinical Psychology Theory, Research and Practice,* Dow Jones-Irwin, Homewood, Illinois.

SUBJECT INDEX

AUTHOR INDEX